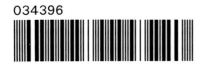

Managing continence

Supporting continence management

a reader for managers

Alice Bradley with Loretto Lambe

RETURN DATE TO BE FOUND
INSIDE BACK COVER

Supporting the Learning Disability Awards Framework
and the Scottish Vocational Qualifications and National
Vocational Qualifications in Health and Social Care

British Library Cataloguing in Publication Data

A CIP record for this book is available from the Public Library

© BILD Publications 2006

BILD Publications is the imprint of:
British Institute of Learning Disabilities
Campion House
Green Street
Kidderminster
Worcestershire DY10 1JL

Telephone: 01562 723010
Fax: 01562 723029
E-mail: enquiries@bild.org.uk

Website: www.bild.org.uk

ISBN 1 904082 84 X

BILD publications are distributed by:
BookSource
50 Cambuslang Road
Glasgow G32 8NB

Telephone: 0845 370 0067
Fax: 0845 370 0068

For a publications catalogue with details of all BILD books and journals telephone 01562 723010, e-mail enquiries@bild.org.uk or visit the BILD website www.bild.org.uk

Printed in the UK by Latimer Trend & Company Ltd, Plymouth

About the British Institute of Learning Disabilities

The British Institute of Learning Disabilities is committed to improving the quality of life for people with a learning disability by involving them and their families in all aspects of our work, working with government and public bodies to achieve full citizenship, undertaking beneficial research and development projects and helping service providers to develop and share good practice.

Acknowledgements

A great many people have helped with the development of this reader. In particular I wish to thank Mary Buchanan, Agnes Forsyth, Caroline Stewart, John Dawson, June Rogers, Rosanne Binnie, Donna Philben, Diane Waugh, David Weir, Michelle Buckley, Trish Fleming, Beryl Sanderson, Andrea Barber, June Rogers, Janet Blanin and Loretto Lambe for their advice and contributions.

About the author

Alice Bradley is a freelance trainer and consultant and an Open University tutor. She has worked with people with learning disabilities of all ages, as well as families and professionals, for many years in schools, urban and rural communities and higher education establishments in the UK and several countries in Asia and Africa. She is currently undertaking work for BILD, the Scottish Consortium for Learning Disability and the Scottish Qualifications Authority. She is the author of many books on learning disabilities.

Contents

Introduction

This book is intended for managers, senior practitioners, carers and professionals concerned with support services for people with learning disabilities who have a specific interest in the topic of continence and who want to continue their professional development. It should also be of interest to support staff members studying for the Learning Disability Awards Framework and the Scottish Vocational Qualifications and National Vocational Qualifications in Health and Social Care.

The book is accompanied by an easy-read booklet for people with a learning disability, *Everybody Needs Toilets*, and a workbook for support workers and carers, *Helping People with Learning Disabilities Manage Continence.*

The purpose of the reader is to explore the issues surrounding the management of continence, the support required by people with learning disabilities and the implications for people who work in services and for family carers.

Reasons for writing this book

The first reason for writing this book is that relatively little has been written about continence in relation to people with learning disabilities. In one way this is strange, yet in another it isn't. There's still a considerable amount of silence around the issue of incontinence for the population in general, so why should it be any different for people with learning disabilities? It's true that continence care has begun to attract more public attention over recent years, but change in understanding and better support are slow in coming. Campaigning organisations with a particular interest in continence, such as *In*contact and PromoCon, for example, and continence specialists, have been the prime instigators. There has also been much more government involvement in continence care recently, as well as in the general health care of people with learning disabilities, with an increasing number of policy documents and guidelines being published. This is a considerable advance, undoubtedly, but how much real difference has it made to the support provided to people with learning disabilities and carers? Government policy advocates an integrated approach to continence care which caters for all members of the population. While this is encouraging, there is as yet only limited improvement in the quality of health care services available to people with learning disabilities.

This disparity in the provision of continence services is partly due to the assumption that when someone with a learning disability experiences incontinence it must be as a direct result of their learning disability. Yet the causes of incontinence for most people with learning disabilities are the same as for those in the general population – age-related changes, the menopause, stroke and illness or infection, for example. It is true that the proportion of people with learning disabilities experiencing incontinence is higher than in the population as a whole and that the incidence increases with the severity of the impairment, but the link is by no means straightforward. Incontinence occurs as a result of a whole variety of factors – physiological, psychological, social and environmental. Cognitive ability may well play a part, especially in those with profound and multiple disabilities, but we cannot assume that it is the primary cause in all cases. Several writers (Hyams et al, 1992; Stanley, 1997; Hutchinson, 1998; Rogers, 2001) warn against being too quick to make a causal link between incontinence and cognitive capacity. Hutchinson (1998) highlights the fact that rather than developmental delay being the determining factor, incontinence for many people with learning disabilities is more likely to be caused by things like infection, weak sphincter muscles or emotional upset, all of which are treatable. Rogers, in her ongoing work with disabled children, has shown repeatedly that many children with learning disabilities who are not spontaneously continent by the age of two or three can become so if the right approach is adopted, although probably at a later age. Even within the most severely disabled sector of the population there are many who have achieved at least some degree of continence. Hutchinson (op cit) believes that 'social continence is a realistic option for the majority of people with profound disabilities' (p.9).

Most studies on continence have concentrated on children and usually on behavioural approaches to toilet training. There is a dearth of information on continence management for adolescents or adults with learning disabilities. Much more research is required and it is hoped that some additional work might be stimulated as a result of this publication. Research on toilet training in childhood is useful, not least because it reminds us that we need to take account of past history and its possible effects when we consider the likely causes of incontinence in adolescence and adulthood. But it has its limitations in relation to continence management across the lifespan. The focus in this reader is on continence management with and for adolescents and adults, rather than children, because the issues are different, although there is some overlap. The issues discussed in the book are relevant to people supported at home and by different types of support services, and day, residential and supported living.

When I was interviewing people for this book, some said, 'Oh, continence – that's about toilet training, isn't it?' Well, it is to an extent – but it's about much more than just that. For a start, 'training' implies something that is done *to* people, whereas 'continence management' takes a much broader perspective and encompasses a wider range of activities than just using a toilet. The term is more comprehensive and includes support as well as needs. The nature of this support will vary widely, not only in relation to the individuality of each of the heterogeneous groups of people who have learning disabilities, but also according to individual circumstances and the cause and type of an individual person's continence difficulties. Thus, the self-management of continence can range from assessment, diagnosis and cure of an underlying physical cause with the full involvement and consent of people able to express themselves verbally and take quite complex decisions, to the provision of more effective continence aids that improve the quality of life for people with profound and multiple learning disabilities.

A second reason for writing the book is that incontinence disrupts lives and constrains opportunity, not only for the individuals who experience it, but for those who care for and about them, as illustrated by these comments from some mothers I spoke to:

> 'The problem is that up until maybe the age of ten – it may actually be a wee bit more now, up to the age of thirteen – there are products, mainly Dri Nites – they are shaped like a pant, they're not a pad, they're not bulky, they are neat, they don't draw attention to the fact that the child or the young person is wearing an incontinence product, and that's all important too, as I say, our children have enough to bear with without drawing attention to every single one of their problems, and if incontinence is one of their problems, people shouldn't need to know about that. And that's the only product that I know of that is useful to a child of maybe up to twelve, depending on their size. After that, from what I can see, no support is available that isn't big and bulky – a lot of the products are good at what they are designed to do, but they don't take in aesthetics. And I think in some ways that's taking away dignity – a young child, depending on their needs – some of them may not be aware of the fact that they are wearing a product anyway, but some children will be aware of the fact that they don't want to be wearing something that shows they have no control over their own continence.

You probably don't live the life that you should be living, the person isn't being allowed the variety of outings that they would be given under different circumstances, if that is a big problem for you, because you think is it worth putting myself through it? Is it worth putting my daughter through it? And again, you're always having to deal with the public attitude. And public attitude varies so very, very much. I mean, even going back to the fact that my daughter has epilepsy – if my daughter takes a seizure, she could urinate – in that circumstance I've never had any bad help – people have been very helpful and kind – but even just the anxieties for parents, it's just another thing you have to cope with, it's just another area in your life which is wide open to all and sundry. Just basically always having to explain yourself, and explain what's wrong with your child – it's just a feeling of being very exposed.

You feel as if you are going around telling all and sundry about how life is – you have to go over your story about how life with your disabled child is – so many people come in through your door – social workers, carers – and you're constantly having to tell the same story. And basically your life is not your own private life; your home is not your own private home. You feel as if life is being – you don't even go down to the shops with a special needs child without being noticed – everybody notices you. As a carer, as a parent, that varies on my mood – some days I find it quite amusing, and other days, if I feel a bit more sensitive, I can get really quite upset. I've had people moving out of the way to let me by just so they can have a better look at just what the commotion is that's happening behind them. But on the other hand I have come across very, very kind people, so I can't say it's all the one category. There's quite a variety.

I would say the biggest problem is that my son doesn't give me any communication as to when he wants to go. But in saying that, last week I said to Michael, using the sign for the toilet and he got up, he went into the hall, and I said to my mum I have a feeling that he must need the toilet. So I took him in, he hadn't done anything, so I was able to get the nappy off, sit him on the toilet pan, but the only problem was that he didn't sit to do number one, so I managed to get him to do a number two, and I was giving him praise for that, and he can't wipe his bum, so obviously I've got to do that part, and I was disappointed that he had done the toilet on the floor – just a number one. But in saying that, of course, you can't have it all ways. At least doing something himself is a bit of a benefit. When he was in the toilet I said 'Do you want to flush it, M?', so he's like that looking at me as if to say 'What?' So I said 'Push it down.' So I told him to push it down and he did it, and after that I was giving him some praise and he was laughing. So that was sort of promising. He doesn't seem to be doing the toilet in his nappy too much, but he is still wetting himself. So that to me is more of a problem, because you can't judge when they're doing that. My worry is at night-time – sometimes you are going in – I've got a plastic cover on the bed – but even with that, sometimes I can go in and find out the nappy's quite sodden. I don't know if it's because he's going through puberty or not. That might be a problem as well. The biggest worry is actually doing the front part – I really don't know how to work out that part.

I would say, really, nothing's really helped. It's just a matter of guesswork really. Other than getting the continence pads off the doctor and that, that's not so bad, because I was buying my own nappies for a while, up until they couldn't fit him any more. I didn't realise that he was entitled to incontinence pads. Nobody told me. And then it was one day – I think I was talking to someone in the school – and I think it was them who told me I had to be referred to the doctor for it. And then as I went down – I can't remember what you call them, if it was a health worker or whatever, a health visitor maybe, and when I went down to see her she told me – I must have been on file for her to come out and see me, and she hadn't done it. And M was about five before I even went to investigate anything like that. Because I could get pads out of the shops and then I just didn't think I'd be entitled to it. And then you always think, maybe they'll toilet train themself eventually, but eventually you have to go down that road. You have to find out more about incontinence pads and that. So I got the referral, and I think that's when she said – she said, "I'd wondered why you hadn't come down to see me years ago". Now, I wasn't told anything about this. And I just said I'd mentioned it to the school and they'd told me to go and see my own doctor. Then she must have put me down for a referral, and I got to see her, the health visitor, and I said to her 'I was never informed of this'. Just after that – what she did was, she checked up on my son, and what they do is they ask you how many nappies you go through a day, and based on that, basically that is the amount they give you. The school has to get a pack as well. So you are constantly going down and getting them.'

If we can find better ways of providing support for continence management to people with learning disabilities and carers we can perhaps begin to remedy some of the inequalities in the health care support systems and limit the effects of incontinence. At the very least we have a responsibility to respond to the challenges and improve continence care for the people we support.

How the book is organised

There are four chapters:

Chapter 1 **The management of continence** deals with the topic of continence management within the context of recent developments in continence care, government policy and health care initiatives. The main types and causes of continence are explored.

Chapter 2 **The self-management of continence for people with learning disabilities** is about the importance of involving individuals as fully as possible in the management of their own continence. This chapter explores what has been written about continence management and people with learning disabilities, the challenges facing staff in this area of their support work, continence management and touch, and the different types of support that are likely to be required.

Chapter 3 **Encouraging and supporting choice in continence management** covers the issues of choice and decision-making in relation to continence, and the challenges of this for support workers and managers are discussed. Suggestions are given on how managers can encourage and support staff to facilitate choice and decision-making. There is particular emphasis on communication and interaction within the context of choice.

Chapter 4   **Organisational aspects of managing continence** is about organisational responsibilities and policies in relation to the management of continence and their significance for service provision and management. The relevance of care management, duty of care, adult protection and risk management for continence management is explored, as well as support outside the service setting, reporting and recording and the importance of multidisciplinary teamwork.

Each chapter relates to and expands upon a corresponding chapter in the staff workbook. Throughout, information is given and examples drawn from research studies and the first-hand experiences of the advisory and support group whose members contributed to the development of this book and the others in the *Managing Continence* series.

Following chapter 4, there is a resources section that describes the range and use of continence aids currently available and provides information about some of the people, organisations and resources that can help with the management of continence.

Aims of the book

The aims of the book are to:

- highlight issues relevant to managers with particular emphasis upon supporting individuals and staff in the management of continence, eg service responsibilities, policy and procedural guidelines, recording and reporting, government documentation and legislation

- draw upon relevant research studies

- provide background information about the management of continence

- explore current initiatives in continence care

- provide information about useful organisations and resources

- encourage reflection and subsequent action

- raise questions and suggest areas for further investigation and research

Activities and reflections

Throughout the book you are invited to consider how the issues discussed relate to your own service and experience. A series of activities and reflections are provided to enable you to do this. You may find these helpful for other purposes, such as continuing professional development or S/NVQ-related study. They might also be relevant for staff meetings or for staff supervision purposes.

The advisory and support group

The voices of people with learning disabilities, carers, support workers and managers are represented in this publication through the work of the advisory and support group. I met with these people on a regular basis over a period of eight months to draw upon their experience and listen to what they had to say.

Mostly, we met on a one-to-one basis because of the sensitivity of the topic and for practical reasons such as their family responsibilities and distance, but occasionally two or three of us met together. Individuals who used augmentative communication were assisted by a staff member at our discussions. The insights and input of the advisory and support group have been invaluable in constructing this reader and the other books in the pack. These comments from one mother reflect the difficulties families face in everyday life when their relative has continence difficulties.

> 'I think the biggest problem is probably the restrictions it puts on you – like if you go somewhere for the day – you learn over the years to manage things fairly well – everyone has their own ideas about how they would do that, because we're all individuals. You have to find somewhere where your child can actually get lifted, on to a plinth, but usually it is on the floor of a disabled toilet – so you can change their pad, get them cleaned up and make them feel comfortable. That is the biggest problem that I encounter, certainly, that everything has to be meticulously planned and probably timed – you're thinking, well, we can go out for two hours because she will be fairly comfortable for two hours, but then you have to come back home or try and find somewhere.

The same difficulties apply when you're on holiday, when you're out of your own environment. In the long term it's not just something that puts a restriction not only on you as a family, but also on your son or daughter, and the opportunities that they have to do things that other people take for granted, I think.'

Chapter 1

The management of continence

Introduction

Incontinence presents problems for a considerable number of people with learning disabilities and those who support them, yet has received scant attention in both literature and practice. One reason is that incontinence is very much a taboo subject. We might be quite happy to discuss a bad back, or pulled ligament, but we draw the line at something as intimate as bowel or bladder problems. Even the efforts of organisations which campaign for greater public awareness and information, such as *In*contact and PromoCon (details in the resources section of this reader) are only slowly beginning to have an effect on the population as a whole. Internet discussion groups show how strong is the social stigma experienced by people with continence problems. A recent Department of Health publication highlighted not only the health consequences of incontinence, but also the resulting social problems such as bullying in schools and workplaces, restricted opportunities in work, education and leisure, and conflicts within relationships (DoH, 2000a).

People with learning disabilities experience just as much inequality in this area of health care as they do in others. High quality continence support is important for both health and social reasons, and because people with learning disabilities have the same rights as others to the best health care possible. Front-line staff play a crucial role since it is they who are involved on a day-to-day basis with the people requiring assistance with continence management. People with learning disabilities who require support with their intimate care needs are particularly vulnerable to abuse, something discussed in chapter 4 of this reader. Front-line staff are the people most likely to discover or suspect abuse, or to have abuse disclosed to them.

The first chapter in this reader explores continence management within the context of person-centred health care, individual rights and quality of life. If services are to support people in the management of continence, managers and staff have to have a clear understanding of the kinds of problems people might have and the type of specialist support available. But continence support does not take place in isolation. A holistic and person-centred approach is just as important as it is in other areas of support. With these points in mind, the first chapter discusses:

- different types of incontinence

- the main causes of incontinence

- recent developments in continence care and its relevance for people with learning disabilities

Different types of incontinence

The generic term 'incontinence' covers a whole range of bladder and bowel problems, some more familiar to us than others. These include the following:

Stress incontinence	refers to the leakage of urine or faeces when someone coughs, sneezes, laughs or undertakes exertion. The bladder or bowel is unable to handle the increased pressure of the exertion.
Urge incontinence	means a strong desire to urinate or defecate, often without the necessary warning, and the inability to delay urination or evacuation.
Overflow incontinence	is the frequent leakage of urine or faeces from an overfull bladder or rectum.
Reflex incontinence	occurs without any warning and may be due to nerve damage or cognitive impairment.
Frequency	as the word suggests, is the need to urinate more often than is normally expected.
Total incontinence	is the absence of both bladder and bowel control.
Enuresis	means loss of bladder control at night.
Encopresis	describes the lack or loss of bowel control.
Nocturnal encopresis	is loss of bowel control during the night.
Constipation	which is irregular or difficult defecation, is sometimes associated with urinary incontinence and may be a side effect of medication.

People may experience one or more than one type of incontinence at the same time.

The extent of an incontinence problem and its effect on the person concerned can vary considerably depending on circumstances. For example, getting up to go to the toilet once or twice during the night might be considered little more than a nuisance if you can manage everything yourself. However, in Evelyn's case, it is exacerbated by the fact that she has mobility difficulties associated with age and physical impairment. She usually needs to get up only once during the night, occasionally twice. Because she needs help getting to the toilet, she has to press the buzzer and wait for a member of staff. She is finding her increasing dependence distressing, and the need for support from others in this intimate area of life intrusive. She realises it is necessary, but this doesn't make it any easier.

Jason, who has profound and multiple learning disabilities and whose communication is non-verbal, is able to express his need to use the toilet. This is noted in his care plan, together with the procedures for night staff as well as day staff. This prevents his having to wear continence pads at night, which he hates.

Reflection

You might like to think about...

...the differences in the perceptions of the managers, staff and individuals about what constitutes a 'problem' in the management of continence.

...how individuals differ in the way in which they view their own need for support in continence management.

How might you get more of an insight from individuals who use services ? What are the implications of this for the guidance you provide for staff in supporting people with continence management? How might you use this in discussion with individual staff members?

The main causes of incontinence

An understanding of the causes of incontinence doesn't guarantee effective support, but it does make it more likely. Categorising causes can be a helpful way of understanding the factors which contribute to incontinence. Stanley (1997), for example, groups factors contributing to incontinence under the headings of environmental, personal and medical. He impresses upon us the importance of understanding someone's previous experience, especially where incontinence might be a form of challenging behaviour, produced because of impoverished social or physical environments, trauma or abuse.

The categories used in this book are medical, developmental, behavioural, dietary and emotional.

Medical causes of incontinence

The medical causes of incontinence have been well researched, perhaps more so than any other category. This is unsurprising since continence is primarily a medical issue. However, its impact is not only medical but also social and personal. The most common medical causes of incontinence are:

- weakness of the bladder outlet and pelvic floor muscles; for women, this can happen after giving birth or because of changes in hormone levels during the menopause

- in men, prostate problems or the surgical removal of the prostate gland

- conditions that affect the nervous system and the communication between the brain and the bladder or bowel, such as stroke, multiple sclerosis, spina bifida, Parkinson's disease, brain injury and cerebral palsy

- temporary illness such as food poisoning or bacterial infection

- emergency or chronic conditions such as colitis, kidney infection or disease

- epilepsy, arthritis, stroke or diabetes

- age-related conditions such as Alzheimer's

- malformations of the bowel or bladder, some of which are the result of congenital impairment

- side effects of certain medication

- anal irritation or dehydration

People with learning disabilities are as likely as anyone else to experience incontinence for one or more of these reasons.

Developmental causes of incontinence

Developmental problems can be neurological or physical and include:

- underdeveloped urinary or bowel systems

- cognitive difficulties understanding any or all elements of the management of continence, eg the need to use a toilet

- problems in the sensory mechanisms required to send the right messages and take the right action

- problems recognising the sensations of a full bladder or bowel

- difficulties with communication

It's clear that these factors are particularly important for people with learning disabilities, given the range of impairments associated with learning disability, the fact that neurological disability is often accompanied by physical or sensory impairment, that neurological systems are complex and that it is often difficult to identify the exact cause of impairment. The majority of people with learning disabilities have some difficulty with communication, ranging from mild to severe and complex, so communicating their needs is not a straightforward matter. Even when there is no medical cause for incontinence, restricted mobility and sensory impairment, for example, can be significant contributory factors.

Behavioural causes of incontinence

Behavioural causes consist of:

- emotional and psychological conditions that people might experience, eg anxiety, fear or acute distress, which can result in enuresis, encopresis or constipation

- mental health difficulties

- difficulties in communication that can result in attracting attention or expressing emotions through enuresis, encopresis or constipation

- lack of exercise and long periods of inactivity, which are behavioural in origin and self-imposed rather than the result of impairment

Dietary causes of incontinence

Although most people are aware that there is a link between diet and continence, there is often misunderstanding about exactly what this link is. A common misconception, for example, is that cutting down fluid intake can improve urinary continence. In fact this can be harmful as it increases the density of urine and may affect the functioning of the kidneys.

The most common diet-related causes of incontinence are:

- significant changes in diet

- an unbalanced diet, eg too many proteins and not enough carbohydrates

- eating contaminated food

- food allergies

- an inappropriate diet, such as liquidised food

- a diet that is too soft and without enough roughage – it's important to remember, however, that there are some people who can only manage a liquidised diet and that non-oral diets do not have roughage; staff are more likely to need specialist support with people whose continence difficulties are related to either of these factors; family members who have been dealing with the problems throughout their relative's lifetime are an invaluable source of support and advice

- inadequate fluid intake

- lack of dietary fibre

Emotional causes of incontinence

Often, incontinence occurs as a result of the physical, psychological or social environments surrounding the person, or that he or she has experienced in the past. These create emotional stress, caused by fear, anxiety or worry, for example. Emotional causes can also be the result of:

- being ignored or neglected

- physical restraint and punishment

- physical, sexual or institutional abuse

- communication difficulties that render people unable to communicate both positive and negative emotions

Incontinence can also be caused by lack of opportunity to learn, as in Sabina's case.

> Sabina has Down's syndrome and severe learning disabilities and is described as having 'no communication or comprehension skills'. She was twenty-four and had recently moved to the UK when this story began. She was incontinent both day and night, wore all-in-one pads and was never encouraged to use the toilet as her family had been told she would always be dependent on them for her basic needs.
>
> A full continence assessment showed that Sabina's incontinence was possibly due to lack of training, and a daily bladder programme was introduced. This included verbal praise and ignoring incontinence. There was significant improvement, Sabina started to express her wishes by means of facial expression and intonation, and refused to wear pads, preferring ordinary underwear.
>
> (Earnshaw and Betts, 2001)

Reflection

You might like to think about...

...the extent to which these causes are relevant to the people in your service.

...how aware support staff in your service are of the causes of incontinence other than medical or the contribution of the impairment.

...the myths that surround the causes of incontinence in your service.

These might be useful issues for staff discussion or supervision.

Recent developments in continence care

Whatever the cause, incontinence has a significant effect on people's lives. Over recent years, campaigning organisations, health professionals and government bodies have invested considerable effort in raising awareness of continence as a health issue and providing better support for those affected by incontinence. *In*contact, a consumer-led organisation committed to raising public awareness and providing information and support to people with bowel and bladder problems, says:

> 'Our vision is a future where incontinence is no longer taboo, where people with bladder and bowel problems have free access to information and support and to the treatments, products and services they need.' (www.incontact.org)

There has been an increasing amount of government guidance available on good practice in continence care over recent years. One of the most helpful publications is *Essence of Care: Benchmarks for Continence and Bladder and Bowel Care*. Produced by the DoH in 2001, this document identifies the factors that constitute best practice, provides a series of benchmarks and lists a number of indicators for each of the factors listed. For example, under *Factor 11, User involvement in service delivery*, the following indicators of good practice are listed:

- 'methods to secure user involvement, eg focus groups, user forums, patients' council, etc to include considerations of religious, cultural, language and age-related and special needs issues

- patients' satisfactions with continence services ... and ... any complaints are addressed

- there is evidence of inter-agency involvement and networking with all stakeholders

- strategies are used to involve users from isolated or hard-to-reach communities'

  (DoH, 2001a)

All factors identified provide detailed information on how that specific aspect of continence care should be delivered. This document is particularly useful to managers seeking to improve continence management in their service as it contains a highly detailed analysis of good practice and provides information on the kind of support that should be made available to all individuals, including people with learning disabilities.

Quality Indicators, Learning Disabilities (NHS Scotland, 2004) provides a framework for assessing the quality of health services available to children and adults with learning disabilities in Scotland. Although not dealing specifically with continence, the publication contains many items that have relevance, such as ensuring involvement and access to the same services as other people, providing information in accessible formats, implementing multidisciplinary practice, providing workforce training and upholding the right of people with learning disabilities to health care screening and appropriate treatment. Like *Essence of Care: Benchmarks for Continence and Bladder and Bowel Care*, the document is a useful one for providing detailed guidelines for managers.

The guidelines described above also provide leverage when people are experiencing discrimination in continence services, especially since the importance of 'prompt, high quality, comprehensive continence services' for everyone is emphasised in the central government publication, *Good Practice in Continence Services* (DoH, 2000a). The model of good practice presented advocates with an integrated approach to identification, assessment and appropriate treatment. The impact of incontinence is highlighted, eg people with continence problems are frequently embarrassed and ashamed, keep their condition hidden, are reluctant to seek assistance and are unaware of the help available to cure or manage their incontinence. One of the most important sections is that dealing with assessment, since it pinpoints the level of service people are entitled to. This section begins, 'All patients presenting with incontinence should be offered an initial assessment by a suitably trained individual' (p.12) and then identifies the key components of such an assessment. Once the assessment is completed, a management/treatment plan should be discussed, agreed and a copy given to the person concerned. A list of treatment options is provided, eg general advice on healthy living, bladder training, improved mobility, improved access to toilets, pelvic floor and sphincter exercises, review of medication, provision of continence aids and more specialist support and intervention. This section has particular relevance for people with learning disabilities who are often automatically issued with incontinence pads rather than having their symptoms investigated. Hutchinson (op cit), for example, writes of a woman with learning disabilities who was assessed by a district nurse as having a mixture of stress and urge incontinence. She was immediately provided with incontinence pads rather than being offered treatment options. When the nurse's actions were challenged, the woman was given electrotherapy and medication which resolved her continence problem and saved her wearing pads unnecessarily for the rest of her life.

Commenting on the guidelines *Good Practice in Continence Services* (op cit), Thomas (2000) points out that services should cover prevention as well as treatment and management, apply to faecal as well as urinary incontinence and to children as well as adults. Foremost responsibility for continence care is with the primary care team. People who have hitherto been lowest on the care agenda, including those who have learning disabilities, are mentioned specifically in the guidelines. In current practice, Thomas asserts, people with continence problems may be assessed but are unlikely to receive comprehensive management plans that follow an agreed care pathway, despite the fact that their continence problem might have a simple solution. She contends that current government policy will require a change of attitude for many nurses since the previous response of containment is no longer acceptable on its own.

The value of these documents to service managers is that they provide information about the quality of continence care that should be available to people with learning disabilities just as much as to everyone else and that they identify standards for good practice. The detailed information that is presented in *Essence of Care: Benchmarks for Continence and Bladder and Bowel Care* is particularly useful in relation to policy development within services and the provision of more detailed guidelines for staff members supporting individuals with continence management.

ACTIVITY 1: **Using documents in staff training and development**

Download and look at the publication, *Essence of Care: Benchmarks for Continence and Bladder and Bowel Care* (op cit) which is available on the website www.publications.doh.gov.uk/essenceofcare

Think about how you might use it in training or discussion sessions with staff (individuals or a group) and jot down some ideas to try out.

Documents can be useful, not least because they inform you about policy and entitlement. Having access to a local specialist, however, is essential. The first port of call should be the local continence adviser as they are the expert in this area of health care, can arrange assessments and appropriate treatment, provide information and advice and enable people to obtain the necessary products and equipment.

Continence care and people with learning disabilities

Despite the increased emphasis on continence care, people with learning disabilities continue to experience inequality in this area of health care, just as they do in others. There is a considerable amount of misinformation around, including the assumption discussed earlier that any incontinence is a direct consequence of the learning disability and that continence aids are the only answer. Continence pads are often supplied as a matter of course, rather than symptoms investigated and appropriate treatment provided, as would happen with non-disabled people. Rogers (2002) found that the vast majority of paediatric assessments undertaken in a number of continence services across England were 'no more than a free nappy/pad assessment form with questions relating to the degree of wetting and soiling and the number or type of products to be issued' (p.958). Underlying problems that might cause or contribute to incontinence were often not explored because most health professionals believed the incontinence to be due to the learning disability. Too many children, Rogers believes, are labelled as incontinent too soon and no further effort is made to help them to become continent. Similarly, Rigby (2001) contends that assessments have long been used as 'pad assessments and seen predominantly as a route to product provision rather than a way of identifying and perhaps treating problems' (p.49).

If health professionals operate according to such assumptions, it is unsurprising that parents and teachers often have incorrect or incomplete information. Rogers (op cit) found a considerable lack of knowledge among teachers about the causes, management and treatment of incontinence in children, with many thinking that there might be a behavioural element to children's incontinence, such as attention seeking or laziness and failing to look any further for possible alternative causes.

Another reason for unequal treatment is that many generic health professionals have difficulties communicating with people who have learning disabilities. This is compounded by the tendency to treat people as a homogeneous group rather than individuals with specific needs. Comments from two people with learning disabilities indicate the extent of their frustrations with this practice. In the NHS Health Scotland (2004) *Health Needs Assessment Report: People with Learning Disabilities in Scotland*, White says, 'Health professionals need to try to understand that not everyone has the same needs. I also feel that GPs do not always understand the person's feelings even if they are told them' (p.iii). In the same report, Wallace agrees, 'I think that it is important for the NHS to improve the health of people with learning difficulties because we are as important as anybody else and should have the same rights and opportunities to access services. Professionals should listen to people with learning difficulties because we are the experts. We know what our bodies need and require. It might take longer to know what is wrong with us but you have to be patient' (NHS Scotland, 2004, p.iii).

Signposts for Success in Commissioning and Providing Health Services for People with Learning Disabilities (DoH, 1998) was produced to help combat the problems health professionals have in responding to, and providing treatment for, people with learning disabilities. Based on the views of over 500 people with learning disabilities, family carers, professionals and support services, this publication identifies several prerequisites for good practice in the provision of health care, including: the recognition of rights, the provision of information in appropriate formats, positive attitudes, good communication skills, consent and flexibility. *Once a Day* (DoH, 1999b) has a similar purpose. Designed for primary health care teams, including both medical and administrative staff, its purpose is 'To promote good practice in enabling people with learning disabilities to access and receive good quality services from primary health care teams' (p.2). The publication is constructed around salient information about learning disability and pinpoints health care inequalities. It includes comments from people with a learning disability and their relatives, scenarios for discussion and examples of good practice and is user friendly.

The White Paper, *Valuing People* (DoH, 2001b) and the Scottish Executive review of services for people with learning disabilities, *The same as you?* (2000), both stress the need for better health care services for people with learning disabilities. Health Action Plans, advocated in *Valuing People*, provide one mechanism for helping people achieve them. The Department of Health intends that all young people and adults in England who have learning disabilities should have a Health Action Plan, compiled by the person concerned with help from a health worker and others who provide support. The plan should detail actions that will enable the individual to have a healthy life, such as getting the right information in an accessible format, having regular check-ups and living a healthy lifestyle. Continence is specified as one of the areas for inclusion when necessary. *Valuing People* also identifies the need for professionals to act as 'health facilitators' if the health inequalities experienced by people with learning disabilities are to be overcome. Primary care is generally the first point of contact for health care, but people with learning disabilities often encounter difficulties in obtaining the right kinds of services, so require particular support. Mobbs et al (2002) believe that, because of their health-based training and specialist skills in working with people with learning disabilities, community learning disability nurses are particularly suited to the role of health facilitator. They point out that many nurses are already actively involved in health promotion and health surveillance schemes for people with learning disabilities, as discussed in *Health of the Nation* (DOH, 1995).

Corbett et al (2003) identify some of the factors which impede access to better health care for people with learning disabilities. These include difficulty knowing when to seek advice, difficulty understanding available information and problems with transport to attend appointments. The issue of consent is a difficult one for support staff and health care professionals alike, especially if these same people are also expected to help individuals reach decisions. Corbett et al consider health facilitation as a role for everyone supporting the person, family and paid carers as well as health professionals. However, based on studies in North Staffordshire and Wolverhampton, they also believe that it is necessary to have designated health facilitator posts, since 'if this role is added to that of current members of community learning disability teams, rather than to a designated post, the impact on the general health of people with learning disabilities would continue to be undermined because of other commitments and priorities' (p.409). Not only would people with learning disabilities benefit from improved health facilitation, in terms of better support and increased awareness of need, the allocation of more time for procedures to be explained and better informed primary, acute, secondary and specialist health care teams, but specialist services and GP practices would increase their knowledge of the numbers of people with learning disabilities under their care.

The same as you? advocates the development of personal life plans for people with learning disabilities in Scotland. Regular assessments of their health needs and plans of care should be included as integral components, as outlined in *Promoting Health, Supporting Inclusion* (NHS Scotland, 2002). The *Health Needs Assessment Report: People with Learning Disabilities in Scotland* (NHS Scotland, 2004) asserts that barriers account for only some of the problems people with learning disabilities face in accessing services and supports for their health needs. Among other factors that impede access are past experiences, social disadvantage, inequalities within society and lack of training for health professionals. For example, 87 per cent of GPs in Glasgow reported that they were unaware of the health needs of their patients with learning disabilities, 83 per cent thought health screening should be available to these patients but only 15 per cent thought it should be provided by the GP or practice nurse (NHS Scotland, 2004). The report contains recommendations to reduce health inequalities and promote social inclusion, and identifies five areas that require specific action if the health of people with learning disabilities is to improve and inequalities be reduced. These are:

- leadership and accountability (which include strategies for health improvement)

- infrastructure (development, planning and monitoring)

- specific interventions (including health screening)

- information

- education

The document says, 'We need a workforce that knows about the needs of people with learning disabilities, is not afraid of disability, treats people with respect, and works in partnership with persons with disabilities, family carers and with other professions' (p.98). This has considerable significance for the management of continence.

Reflection

You might like to think about...

...how the five areas that require specific action outlined above are relevant to the management of continence in your own service and your own local area.

...how, for continence management, your service rates in terms of leadership (your own role), accountability, planning and monitoring, and information.

...what you think could be done better.

Concluding comments

The exploration of the causes and types of incontinence and recent developments in continence care, explored in this opening chapter, provides the context for the topics in the remainder of the book. People with learning disabilities experience inequality in all areas of health care, including continence. Collaboration between professionals, in both mainstream and specialist services, people with learning disabilities and family carers is essential if we are to change this. There is a commitment in several quarters to move forward, backed up by government initiatives, such as those referred to above. We have a responsibility to capitalise on this.

In this chapter I have identified several issues I believe have significance for effective continence management. In summary, these are:

- the right of people with learning disabilities to equal treatment in continence care

- the importance of understanding continence within a framework of holistic health care support

- the need for staff and managers to understand about types and possible causes of incontinence

- the need for a more comprehensive and co-ordinated approach to continence management within services, with support from specialist health professionals

- the right of the person with learning disabilities to be involved in the management of their continence

These points lead on to a fuller discussion of how we can provide better support for people with learning disabilities, which is developed throughout the remainder of the book. One mother summed this up by stressing the need for change, both in the perceptions of others and in public facilities:

> 'I think more people have to be made more aware of the fact that many people in wheelchairs are incontinent and wouldn't be capable of using a public toilet. I think it's a misconception that the vast majority of the public think people in wheelchairs can use a disabled toilet. So that's something that needs to be examined quite closely – why is this? What are our perceptions of people that are using wheelchairs? Do they just make the assumption all the time that it's someone who's like you or me, but sitting in a wheelchair and they can't walk? Let's raise awareness about learning disability, about people with sensory impairment, that prevents them managing, perhaps, their own continence. And let's look at what needs to happen, in public disabled toilets, but also in places like hotels, like supermarkets, big stores – all that kind of thing – libraries, places where ordinary people, actually, every day, think nothing about

"Oh, my goodness, I need to go to the toilet". I think that is something that has to be looked at. Obviously, there's huge cost implications for that, but until organisations can try and justify it – and whether that's gathering statistics in the first instance of how many people using wheelchairs would be unable to manage their own continence in the Glasgow area, for example. So a first step might be looking statistically at the numbers – and I can tell you right now that they will be high, really high – so that has to be the justification, surely, looking at social inclusion policy, and starting with that – how can they implement social inclusion policies if people can't access things that other people can access because of toilet needs?'

Chapter 2

The self-management of continence for people with learning disabilities

Introduction

People with learning disabilities experience incontinence for the same sorts of reasons as everyone else, eg conditions associated with ageing, such as stroke or decreased mobility, medical conditions such as diabetes and epilepsy, factors affecting women's health, including menstruation, childbirth and the menopause, physical impairment, and men's health issues, such as prostate problems. The learning disability might play a part, especially when the person has profound and multiple disabilities and complex health needs, but is by no means the only factor to consider. Incontinence can be temporary, such as after certain kinds of surgery, or more permanent.

There isn't a great deal written about continence management and people with learning disabilities. Much of the literature is about toilet training, usually with children. This is understandable as the attainment of continence in childhood can prevent all sorts of problems in adult life, both for the individual concerned and for family carers and service staff. But it leaves considerable gaps in our knowledge about the broader question of effective continence management for adolescents and adults. One thing we do know is that active involvement of the person concerned and, where appropriate, family carers, is as important in continence management as in other areas of practice.

This chapter includes information about:

- studies of continence management and people with learning disabilities

- the challenges facing staff supporting people with continence management

- continence management and touch

- the 'self-management of continence' and what it means for people with learning disabilities and those who support them

- the range of support that might be required

People with learning disabilities and continence management

Most research on continence and learning disabilities has concentrated on toilet training for children, although some involves adolescents and adults. Methods have been predominantly behavioural, with some variation, such as changes in daily routines and lifestyle. Although this is a narrower focus than the one in this book, it is an important element of continence management and can help us towards a better understanding of the attainment of continence.

Huntley and Smith (1999) describe a long-term follow-up of the behavioural treatment of encopresis (lack or loss of bowel control) for adults living in the community, which had utilised high-fibre diets and bulking agents, prompted toileting and positive reinforcement. They found that six of the nine people with severe learning disabilities who were originally treated as teenagers or young adults were free of major soiling accidents over periods ranging from five to 17 years, two were partially free and one had experienced relapse, thought to be at least partly affected by sexual assault. Lancioni et al (2001) report on a review of literature dealing with treatment for encopresis which consisted of environmental and routine changes, eg changes in rising times and increase in toilet visits, medication, adaptations to diets and the use of continence aids, with the emphasis on behavioural treatment such as scheduled toileting, reinforcement, tokens and overcorrection. They found outcomes to be 'fairly encouraging' (p.55).

Smith and Smith (1998) express concern that behavioural approaches to continence training, which have proved successful in the past, are largely ignored today and their impact underrated. In a comprehensive review ranging from the 1960s until the present day, they emphasise the rights of people with learning disabilities to high quality continence care, equal access to investigation and the treatment of their choice by skilled and informed professionals.

Many children with learning disabilities do become fully continent, some between the usual ages of two and four, some later. Roijen et al (2001), for example in a study of 601 children and adolescents with cerebral palsy in the Netherlands, found that 38 per cent of this group who also had learning disabilities were dry by the age of six. One thing we do know is that the more severe the impairment, the higher the likelihood of incontinence. People who have both physical impairment and profound intellectual impairment are among those most likely to be incontinent. In a cohort of 105 young adults living in the community in northern Finland, Von Wendt et al (1990) found that 94 per cent of those with mild disabilities were continent by day and night but only 21 per cent of those with profound disabilities were. Smith and Smith (1998) tell us that around a quarter of people with profound learning disabilities acquire urinary continence and almost half acquire bowel control. Several writers (McNeal et al, 1983; Rogers, 2001; Roijen et al, 2001) identify various factors associated with the attainment of continence, which include age, the socialisation of the child, maturation of the neurological system, bilateral involvement, communication skills and mobility. It's clear that problems in one or more of these areas can contribute to incontinence for people with profound and multiple disabilities. A considerable number of children with profound learning disabilities do attain full continence, with or without specialist intervention and support, although these are more likely to be those children who do not have complex additional impairments or health needs. Lancioni et al (op cit), while reporting in their literature review on the treatment of encopresis that failures were only reported with people with severe and profound learning disabilities, say nevertheless, 'The fact that some other people with a low level of functioning were successful in acquiring a satisfactory performance ... would exclude a direct link between level of functioning and outcome' (p.55).

Stanley (1997) adopts a broader perspective in his study of continence, highlighting the importance of social considerations and of finding more valued forms of continence management. Continence is a complex set of skills so we need to be aware of possible contributory factors, in addition to the learning disability, and fully informed about how disabled people acquire continence, if we are to provide effective support. Medical or biological causes, low levels of social interaction, abuse and neglect can all play a part. Incontinence may be a learned response to an inappropriate environment, a communicative act or a response to emotional trauma. As long ago as 1963, Ellis found that, while damage to the central nervous system might have contributed to incontinence for people with learning disabilities in a long-stay institution, the major reasons were low staff expectations and few opportunities for learning. Since many of those using adult services today have lived in institutions, this has obvious relevance for continence management within services (Earnshaw and Betts, 2001).

The challenges facing services in the management of continence

Services are most effective in helping people manage continence when managers and support workers have a clear idea of what kind of support is required, are conversant with individuals' previous history, informed about the specialist help available and prepared to spend time helping people find the solution that is right for them as individuals. Better continence management is crucial for the people concerned and, where relevant, for family carers, but is also important for staff. In a study of intimate and personal care provision for people with profound and multiple intellectual disabilities, Carnaby and Cambridge (2002) found that staff most disliked tasks such as washing people's genitalia, changing continence pads, giving enemas and cleaning up bodily fluids. Support workers interviewed felt undervalued, were disheartened at the lack of support and recognition by managers of the importance of personal and intimate care, and were concerned that they were left to develop their own criteria for good practice. Guidance was too generic, they reported, and did not address critical issues such as adult protection and the diversity and complexity of the tasks involved in intimate care. As a result of their study the authors produced the training pack, *Making it Personal: Providing Intimate and Personal Care for People with Learning Disabilities* (Cambridge and Carnaby, 2000), designed to tackle some of these issues.

With the closure of long-stay hospitals and increasing life expectancy, services are now more likely to provide for growing numbers of people with profound and multiple disabilities and complex health needs. Since these are the people most likely to have continence problems, better continence management in services is becoming increasingly important. Mansell et al (2002), studying 500 small homes in England, found that a high proportion of people who use services had significant support needs, that a quarter of those surveyed could not walk alone and three-quarters had what were described as 'toilet accidents'. Over 30 per cent were described as non-verbal or nearly so and nearly half had challenging behaviours. These findings have particular implications for staff training, something that is discussed in chapters 3 and 4.

It is important to bear in mind the fact that the vast majority of people with learning disabilities have always lived with their families. Although more adults are moving into their own accommodation, usually with some kind of support, many will continue to live with their parents or, in some instances, other family carers. People with profound and multiple learning disabilities are more likely to live in the family home well into adulthood and often for life. Family carers know their relative best and should be consulted and involved as partners in any continence management plans.

Continence management and touch

Support with continence and other aspects of intimate care involves a level of physical contact that is unusual in other support work. There is a vast difference, for example, in providing physical support to someone who has difficulties walking and assisting the same person with genital hygiene. This is an issue that is very seldom made explicit in job descriptions, interviews or day-to-day practice. Twigg (1998) highlights the culture of silence that surrounds intimate care. We live in a largely non-tactile society and intimate care is something that isn't talked about, is demeaning both to care givers and those receiving care and for which clear practice guidelines seldom exist, other than technical ones. It involves things people would normally do for themselves – touching, which crosses social and personal boundaries, and the social ambiguities associated with touch. There is a tendency for staff to distance themselves from continence care by discussing something else while involved in the task and by getting it over with as quickly as possible.

Touch is also subject to cultural variations. All cultures have strict rules about touch which, if broken, can constitute violation. In such sensitive situations, it's crucial that cultural norms and requirements are known about and people's preferences respected.

In services where all or most staff are white, the implications of touch for individuals from other ethnic groups are not always understood. This doesn't only apply to opposite sex touching, but also to areas of the body that are considered sacrosanct in some religions. In continence management there is obviously a need for a considerable amount of physical contact, so this can create problems if staff are unaware of the cultural and religious practices of particular ethnic groups. Other cultural considerations can create difficulties for people who use services and their families, eg the way in which certain tasks, such as bathing, are undertaken, and religious requirements for washing certain areas of the body. For example:

- Physical contact between sexes may not be acceptable but same sex physical contact may be more common than in western culture.

- Touching certain parts of the body is unacceptable in certain cultures, eg the head, while in others, touching other parts, eg the feet, is a sign of respect.

- Physical contact acceptable in white British culture is invasive in others.

- Body proximity differs from culture to culture and the western concept of personal space is unrecognised in some cultures.

(Bradley, 2002)

The question of touch can be a difficult one for support workers, not only for the reasons mentioned above, but also because there are wide variations in the way individuals feel about and use touch, some of which stems from upbringing and previous experiences. For someone who has been abused, physically or sexually for example, touch may have particular implications. Clearly, there is a need for great sensitivity when exploring issues relating to touch in staff training sessions and in supervision. Equally, training in continence management must take account of the other issues discussed above, especially cultural considerations: equality, discrimination, stereotyping and relationships with people who use services, their families and the local community.

The self-management of continence for people with learning disabilities

Active involvement for people with learning disabilities and more control over their own lives are common themes in today's services. Underpinning these service aspirations are basic principles and values, such as respect, self-determination and autonomy, recognition of diversity and the promotion of individual rights. Self-management is based on these principles, but also incorporates the support people might require.

It is important at this point to stress that 'self-management' has a wide range of interpretations. Some people may need only verbal support and opportunities to access advice and information, such as help in visiting a continence adviser or in finding out about different continence products. Others will need more intense and sustained support. Some people with profound and multiple learning disabilities may not be able to take active control of their continence management and may need total help. However, they will be able to communicate their feelings – of distress, comfort or discomfort, how secure they feel and how relaxed – through sounds, body movements (muscle tensing or relaxing, for instance) and facial expressions. If workers respond sensitively and appropriately, this enables the service user concerned to exercise some control over the management of their own continence support. By providing different experiences (using scents, touch, massage, for example) and trying different ways of doing things (different times of the day, pacing things differently, allowing more time, finding out the person's preferences for different members of staff) workers are providing opportunities for choice. Here again, family carers are the most valuable source of information on what their relatives do and do not like and on how they prefer to be supported. Self-management may be different in nature for people with profound and multiple learning disabilities and for people with less severe learning disabilities, but the principles remain the same: dignity, privacy, respect, choice and the same quality of support, geared towards an individual's specific needs.

One mother told me:

> 'It's looking at attitude to other people and how much you respect them, the amount of dignity that you would expect, things like personal care, modesty. Imagine if this was a relative of yours, or imagine that this is you – trying to put yourself in the other person's shoes – and think how you would feel if you were in this situation. I think most people can relate it to, like, being in hospital for an operation, having to have a bed bath and that kind of thing – I would always remind people – how did you feel when that happened? Or when someone made a personal remark? Always think that although this person may not be able to communicate verbally and might not even be able to show any level of understanding of what's going on round about them, you just don't know, you can never be 100 per cent sure – but even so, you have to remember how would I like to be treated in this situation? And I think that's really, really important. I've often heard remarks bandied about, particularly in hospitals, where people become a bit desensitised, a lot of remarks about personal care, so I would always remind people of that all the time – do you remember a nurse making a remark to you, or making a remark about someone else that you thought was quite offensive? Don't ever fall into that category. And also, although I think it's not a part of the job that I think anybody particularly enjoys, personal care, because you are always aware of embarrassment, of someone else being in a vulnerable situation, I think that you really have to look carefully at how you manage that for the sake of the other person's dignity.'

What does the self-management of continence mean?

At first glance it might seem that 'self-management' in this context is a misnomer. After all, many of the people we are talking about are those with the most severe and complex disabilities, who depend on other people for many aspects of their daily lives. However, 'self-management' has myriad interpretations. Maureen, for example, who has cerebral palsy, has gradually found it more and more difficult to move around as she's got older. She uses a Zimmer frame but doesn't always make it to the toilet on time. Her sphincter muscles have also become weaker. She has a mixture of stress and urge incontinence. Although she speaks, her voice is weak and she also has difficulty with articulation, so it can be difficult to hear her and to make out what she says. She has been used to being independent all her life and looking after her own needs, so she finds it difficult to admit to needing help.

Alison is much younger – 23 in fact. She also has cerebral palsy and cannot move without help. She uses a wheelchair and needs someone to push it for her. She has a profound learning disability and communicates through facial expressions and sounds which are personal to her but which her family and staff in her day centre understand. She wears continence pads and needs almost total help with changing them, eg she can lift her arms a little, taking quite a while to do so, but cannot move her legs or the lower part of her body; she can indicate by nodding her head when she is ready for her trousers, pants and pad to be removed, but cannot help with their removal. Help is provided by her mother at home and centre staff during the day.

Bill lives in a supported living situation and has his own flat. He has a mild learning disability, is diabetic and has epilepsy. He needs to keep a check on his urine but needs help with this. He has recently been prescribed new medication for his epilepsy but there are side effects, which include constipation.

These three people vary considerably in the extent to which they can manage aspects of their own continence and in the level of support they require. Bill requires only limited support – reminders about checking his urine and some degree of help in monitoring and dealing with the effects of his medication. Maureen has greater needs, but can still take a considerable amount of responsibility for managing her own continence. Alison, on the other hand, has more complex needs which require more regular and concentrated support and will, of necessity, be more time-consuming.

Self-management is about a range of things which ensure that the person concerned is involved as much as is possible in their own continence management, depending on their capacity. This means ensuring that the person concerned:

- is involved as much as possible in all aspects of continence management – planning, implementing, monitoring, reviewing and adapting the management plan

- has access to relevant information in accessible formats, eg verbal, written (including easy-read), visual (pictures, photos, symbols, signs, videos) and aural (taped, verbal interpretations)

- is provided with choice, together with the necessary support and opportunity to express preferences

- receives the support, treatment and/or management options, resources and facilities that suits them best

- is encouraged and supported to participate as fully as possible in managing their own continence, in whatever way is possible

Where the person concerned has profound and multiple learning disabilities, a family carer, or an advocate, will take on many of these roles while still ensuring as much control and choice as possible for the person themself.

One member of staff told me how continence management was undertaken in her residential service:

> 'It's all built around, like, a lifestyle plan – you know, not writing it for G or anybody else, but working with them on how they would like to be supported and not how you think they should be. The information that would need to be in there would be the stuff that we need to do to keep G safe and healthy. That's got to be in everybody's support plan – everybody's lifestyle plan. Also, G puts into it what she likes to do, how she likes to be supported with personal care. So both are important, our input and G's input. So the practical help, the physical help, everything is detailed.'

She also spoke of anticipating difficulties to save people distress and enable them to have control:

> 'Like with P who is pretty much non-verbal, so that could have been difficult supporting her around her continence. What she is able to do is use a gesture when she wants to go to the bathroom – or maybe she will say one word that indicates she wants to use the bathroom ... if after a while she hasn't been to the bathroom, it's our responsibility to go and see if she needs to go rather than her sit in distress or discomfort, so I would ask. We always make sure that

through the day there are incontinence pads available and at night times when we're on sleepover we make sure the bathroom lights are on so she is able to go to the toilet by herself. It's all about safety and it's all about good communication.'

Why is self-management important?

The days of doing things *for* people with learning disabilities – or even worse, doing things *to* them are long gone. Or are they? Certainly, the rhetoric is there. We talk about 'person-centredness', empowerment and participation, rather than aims and objectives, 'supporting' people rather than 'training' them. But what happens in practice, especially in less visible areas of service provision, such as continence management? Cambridge and Carnaby (op cit) found that, because staff find intimate care tasks demanding and view them negatively, they do things for people and try to get them over as quickly as possible. They describe the 'running commentary' approach some support staff adopt during intimate care, believing that they are involving the person concerned, but in reality just offering information, not necessarily at a pace or in a way that the person can understand and giving no time or opportunity for the person to respond or participate.

I found a similar situation with one staff member I spoke to:

'It's easier to talk to people when you are doing things, it makes it all the easier, and certainly avoid talking about what you are doing, apart from checking I'm not hurting you, is this uncomfortable, is it too hot, too cold? ... because I think the biggest worry is – if you put yourself in their shoes – are they dreading doing this? So if you talk about things that are nothing at all to do with what you are doing it makes it easier sometimes.'

It's easy to see how this approach undermines self-management, but also clear that we cannot expect staff to behave otherwise in an area of work that is generally kept hidden and for which they might receive only limited guidance. Self-management in continence can be empowering for people with learning disabilities, whatever their capacity. It is a time when they can develop better relationships, feel important and valued and develop more control over this private and sensitive area of their lives. It's also a time for listening to people (whether their words or their actions), providing opportunities for choice, learning from them about preferences and perceptions and improving the communication of both partners.

Real participation increases a person's self-esteem and better self-management reduces stigma, increases personal dignity and improves overall quality of life. People who are increasingly able to manage their own continence needs also become less dependent on staff and relatives, which is good for everyone concerned. Earnshaw and Betts (op cit) point to the benefits for services when people attain continence or become more able to manage their own needs: reducing staff workloads, promoting more valued lifestyles, reducing costs and improving care practices.

The type of support people might require

Behind the word 'support' lies great diversity of individual need. Think of Maureen, for instance, mentioned in an earlier example, and what 'support' might mean for her:

- opportunities to express her frustrations and anxieties

- getting information about options

- being supported in arranging a continence assessment (which may or may not identify an underlying medical cause that can be treated)

- having somebody to help her communicate during the assessment

- having treatment or management options explained to her

- being supported in making decisions

Thereafter, support might involve changes to the physical environment, eg having a bedroom closer to the bathroom, a buzzer in her room, a commode for night-time use and possibly pads in case of accidents, all of which would be planned and implemented with her and in accordance with her preferences. There are plenty of opportunities for choice and self-management here.

Support for Alison would be very different, and different again for Bill. Clearly, the starting points for identifying the type of support required are the individual's wants, needs and preferences. This is in stark contrast to the approach which might have been adopted 20 or 30 years ago, where the emphasis would be on a deficit model of ability and identification of the skills in which the person would require training. A holistic approach to continence management starts with the person and the factors that affect their health and well-being. The most obvious vehicle for planning support is the person's care plan (called a support plan in some services, mainly because individuals who use services and staff are unhappy with the dependency implied by 'care', a feeling I share). A support worker I consulted explained how it is done in her service:

> 'The information that would need to be in there would be the stuff to keep S safe and healthy. Also, S would put into it what she likes, how she likes to be supported with her personal care. It's about how people like to be treated but also the practical help, the physical help. Everything is detailed … We're working on all that at the moment, but it takes time.'

Depending on their needs and abilities, people who use services might need support with:

- using toilet facilities, eg help with getting to the toilet, clothing, cleansing themselves

- accessing specialist help, eg from the primary care team, a continence adviser or occupational therapist

- obtaining information in suitable formats, eg easy-read booklets, pictures, symbol-assisted, taped

- finding out about continence aids, eg pads, sheaths, colostomy or ileostomy bags, adaptations for toilets; for example, the Clos-o-Mat is a toilet which washes and dries the genital area of the person using it, thus improving independence and reducing the number of intimate care tasks for staff

- obtaining and using continence aids, eg finding the most suitable, trying out different ones, changing, cleaning and disposing of them

- getting suitable clothing, eg finding suppliers, adapting, buying

- monitoring bodily waste, eg for medical reports, to keep track of certain conditions, to ensure good health and well-being, to monitor the effects of medication

- protecting furniture and bedding, eg chair and bed pads

- personal hygiene, eg preventing smells and stains

Have another look at the list above and you'll notice that many of the supports referred to are about things for workers to do. But a holistic and person-centred approach to helping individuals manage continence care is more than that – it's about how to do it. Support with continence management, perhaps more than any other area of practice requires a high level of sensitivity and awareness. I recall visiting a long-stay hospital in the early eighties where support for continence amounted to nothing more than a conveyor-belt approach to toileting a ward full of women with no regard for individuality, dignity or privacy. The only interaction between staff and residents was the physical contact needed to propel the women into the toilet, remove and replace clothing, assist with cleansing and wash those who had had 'accidents'. Yet it is likely that every one of these women could have managed her own continence given the opportunity to learn to do so. Each one distanced herself from the operation by avoiding eye contact, being completely submissive and making no attempt to participate.

One woman I know told me of the problems she had when she was in hospital:

> 'If I couldn't get there in time, if I had an accident, I had to wait for a long time – an hour – for staff to help me. That made me think I'll just have to do everything for myself.'

More recently, I had occasion to visit another long-stay hospital which is in the process of closing. To use the toilet facilities, I had first to ask for a key and make sure I returned it immediately after use. Toilets were clearly labelled 'Staff' and 'Patients'. I can tell you it didn't give me a great deal of faith in their philosophy or approach!

Applying sensitivity and putting the person at the centre in continence management means that staff must:

- take the lead from the person and do things according to their wishes and preferences

- ensure that the person has enough time and is not rushed, either verbally or by body language

- make sure the person has everything they need

- ensure privacy and avoid unnecessary intrusion

- plan ahead

- make sure toilet facilities are clean and comfortable

- understand and respect cultural requirements

- be sensitive to people's feelings, eg anxiety, fear, embarrassment, guilt

- pace things appropriately

- judge when and when not to intervene

- be prepared to let people make mistakes and take risks

- continually evaluate their own practice

- be flexible, eg try different ways of doing things

One support worker in a multi-occupancy house told me how she tries to approach sensitive issues in a way which won't upset people:

> 'I might say to her I've got a spare ten minutes or so, do you want me to give you a wee shower before you go out – if she hasn't been able to get there on time, I mean. If it's the evening and I'm on sleepover, I'll just say, "I think I'll put my pyjamas on – do you want to put yours on and we can watch TV together?" It's less intrusive than saying, "I think you need to get changed" And she's fine about it.'

Another said:

> 'Everything that's needed is kept in the toilet – everything at hand, so that you're not running around embarrassing people.'

For managers, sensitivity means supporting staff in best practice, which includes:

- being observant and alert to anything that goes wrong and putting it right as soon as possible

- developing effective and sensitive policies and procedural guidelines, monitoring their effectiveness and updating them as required

- creating a service ethos and environment that supports person-centred approaches to continence management

- being there for staff when they need you and showing them that you value their work

- being prepared to join in when necessary

- understanding the demands that continence management places upon staff and being prepared to acknowledge this

- providing the necessary training and support

- leading and encouraging teamwork

Staff also need to be honest about when they need support, as one mother, who is also a professional, pointed out:

> 'Some of the children I have worked with have to be catheterised, and I have been trained to do that, but it would probably more be in a nursing situation. I think if you have a bit of a horror, you have to try not to show that and try and be relaxed and be chatting to the person at the same time. Also, I think if you are not comfortable, I think it's important if you're not comfortable in those situations to take it to your line manager and say, look, I'm really not comfortable and then explore why, why aren't you comfortable? Is it something you can never be comfortable with, is it because you don't feel skilled enough to carry out the procedure, or is it an area you're never going to be comfortable in? I always say to people, if that's not an area you're going to be comfortable in, I think you really need to rethink your job – is this the right area for you to be working in? Because people can sense that you're not comfortable, that you're embarrassed or that you find it distasteful. So rather than hiding it, if you like, there comes a point when you have to say – I just can't do that, and go back to your line manager and re-evaluate what you're doing in that kind of job.'

Reflection

You might like to think about...

...what, in your experience, are the most common types of support people need in relation to the self-management of continence and what kinds of challenge these present for staff and managers.

Concluding comments

Self-management is not about total independence, but about a person-centred approach which incorporates partnership and shared problem solving. In the past we've concentrated too much on 'care', something that is done to or for people and which implies dependency. By changing focus and establishing good working relationships, where we all learn from one another and are open to change, we can improve self-management not for, but with, all individuals who use services, including those with the most profound and multiple learning disabilities. Self-management takes many forms. For people with complex needs it might mean being much more alert to the preferences individuals show through their body movements, facial expressions or the sounds they make, and helping them to use these to influence what happens in the management of their own continence. For those who can advocate for themselves it might mean support with decision-making about different aspects of continence management. Whatever the situation, one of the most important determinants of self-management is choice, which is the subject of the next chapter.

Chapter 3

Encouraging and supporting choice in continence management

Introduction

Pick up any document or textbook about learning disability today and you can be pretty sure choice will feature prominently – which is exactly as it should be. Choices come in all shapes and sizes. Everyday choices, such as what to have to eat, when to go shopping or phone friends or family, are so automatic that we hardly even notice we're making them. This is just as well, as life would become highly stressful if we had to stop and consider every single choice we make. Major decisions are a different matter. Faced with the dilemma of staying in a current job or applying for a new one, of getting married or staying single, of emigrating or staying put, we're only too aware of the complexity of choice-making.

We don't suddenly become adept at making choices. We get lots of practice, right from early childhood, with support and guidance from adults, and more freedom as we get older and become more informed and discerning. Smaller choices with minimal risk give way to more major decisions with much greater possibility for things going wrong. We learn from both right and wrong choices and use the feedback to help us develop competence for future choice-making. It's a cumulative and variable process rather than a foolproof learning experience; we all make wrong decisions pretty regularly throughout life.

Choice can be complex and demanding. Sometimes it feels as if it would be easier to leave it up to someone else. However, if your ability or mine to make choices were taken away suddenly, or if we were deprived of the right to choose, we would be less than happy. This is precisely what has happened to many people with learning disabilities, so it's not surprising that they can find choice confusing.

Choice is just as important in continence management as in other areas of life. But, as Cambridge and Carnaby (op cit) stress, intimate care – which includes continence – is often done *for* or *to* people, with little or no opportunity for them to assert themselves or indicate preferences. Continence management presents an ideal opportunity to encourage and support choice, since many of the elements for making choices are present intrinsically in the activities involved in continence management. In this chapter I explore:

- the reasons why choice is important in continence management

- why choice can be difficult for people with learning disabilities

- ways in which staff can encourage and support choice

- the manager's role in helping staff encourage and support choice

Why choice is important in continence management

Choice is about individuality, personal freedom and autonomy. The White Paper, *Valuing People* (op cit) identifies as one of its objectives:

> 'To enable people with learning disabilities to have as much choice and control as possible over their lives through advocacy and a person-centred approach to planning the services they need.' (p.124)

This includes, among other things, full and active involvement in all decisions affecting their lives and personal well-being.

O'Brien (1987) identified choice as one of the five accomplishments services should pursue, and which subsequently influenced service direction in the UK and elsewhere. The Learning Disability Awards Framework (LDAF) unit, Helping Service Users to Manage Continence, which some of your staff might be studying, includes the importance of encouraging choice and self-management as one of its learning outcomes.

Control over our own bodies is a basic human right. When else could personal choice be more important? Earnshaw and Betts (op cit) highlight the importance of ensuring that interventions in continence management are personal to individuals. Health action plans, introduced in *Valuing People* (op cit) as a means of promoting equal access to health care for people with learning disabilities, identify individual needs and preferences as the cornerstone of good practice. Bodily functions, along with sexual preference and activity, are probably the most personal areas of our lives, ones in which few of us would voluntarily invite the involvement of other people. But all too often, when people require intimate care support, their bodies somehow cease to be their own and activities that would otherwise be carried out in private come into the more public domain.

Choice is vital in continence care but it's easy to forget this. For one thing, continence is often considered less important than other areas of life and incontinence as something that shouldn't be talked about. As a result, not only do things remain static, and new ways of providing support remain unexplored, but opportunities for people to be actively involved in, and make choices about, this very fundamental area of their lives are missed. When we provide opportunities for choice, listen to preferences or help someone act on a decision, we affirm their value and importance. We show that we respect their decisions and their right to control over their own lives. We act as facilitators, not decision-makers. Choice empowers people. The more practice people with learning disabilities have at making choices and the more their choices are listened to and acted upon, the more skilled they become.

This is ably demonstrated by the self-advocacy movement in the UK and worldwide, by means of which thousands of people with learning disabilities have proved their critics wrong, shown that their choices and decisions are as valid as anyone else's and exercised their human rights. Choice in continence management enables people to have a greater say over what happens to their own bodies. Enabling people to understand choice can also help guard against abuse by making them aware of what choices are available to them and encouraging them to say no in potentially abusive situations, or to report concerns. Consent is a highly contentious and challenging issue in support work and is discussed in chapter 4. Encouraging and supporting choice in all areas of life is essential for duty of care responsibilities within services.

Why choice can be difficult

Choice is a complex concept, with considerable room for confusion. Choice-making can often be a particularly difficult process for people with learning disabilities, for a variety of reasons, not just ability. Harris (2003) takes issue with the emphasis on intellectual capacity in choice-making to the exclusion of the social and environmental factors which exert an influence in real life situations. In everyday life, he points out, choice-making is influenced by a number of environmental, social, psychological and personal factors. He advocates a sociological perspective on choice, rather than one focusing solely on a concept of capacity which draws upon 'an idealised sequence of mental activities which are presumed to underpin choice-making' (p.5). His preferred approach takes account of environmental factors, staff behaviour and experiences of choice-making and has particular significance for people with learning disabilities, since many require support with choice and are particularly likely to be influenced by those closest to them whether they be family members or support workers.

Range and diversity are relevant to choice. It can be fairly easy to help people make simple choices, such as which drink to have, but the complexity of more major choices can be off-putting. Obviously, the choices that people need to make about continence are not as significant as some other choices in life – such as where to live – but they are nonetheless important and can affect comfort, well-being and health, as well as personal identity, social relationships and self-worth. Nor is choice a 'once-and-for-all' activity. Needs, personal circumstances and possibilities change, so new choices become necessary and possible.

Harris (op cit) stresses the importance of distinguishing between the process of making a choice, the action of communicating the decision and considering the range of options available. Discussing practical implications, he emphasises the crucial role of the social contexts within which people with learning disabilities make choices and the importance of facilitating choice through:

- organising the environment, eg by providing contextual clues for different options such as colour coding objects

- discussing options and possible outcomes, and the use of natural opportunities presented through routine activities

- providing graduated experiences for choice-making where enough time, support and practice is given to enable people to make choices

Cambridge and Carnaby (op cit) stress the importance of 'helpful' environments where support, social contact and relationships facilitate participation. Person-centred planning places choice within the context of social support, emphasising the importance of maximising connections between people and joint approaches to problem solving. Similarly, in the approach known as 'active support', social and environmental support factors are integral components of choice and decision-making.

This much broader perspective on choice and decision-making is important in continence management, especially for people with more severe and complex learning disabilities. It places choice within a more natural and realistic context rather than abstracting it as a theorised intellectual process. None of us lives in a social vacuum. We are all influenced by the people around us and our personal circumstances when considering our options, so why should people with learning disabilities be any different? At the same time, we need to be aware of the subtle influences we might unwittingly exert on the people we support, such as asking leading questions or showing social disapproval. And we need to recognise that people are even more disempowered by having their decisions listened to but ignored. The critical factor is the extent to which we facilitate choice rather than impose our own decisions. This takes skill, knowledge and understanding and has particular significance for managers whose own understanding of the process of choice and the factors influencing it will have a direct effect on the way in which they provide support for workers.

Reflection

You might like to think about...

...some of the people in your service who have difficulty with choice and what causes them the biggest problem.

...how you might help staff to find ways of overcoming these problems.

Ways of encouraging and supporting choice

If staff are to support choice with continence management rather than imposing their own ideas, they have to:

- be aware of the range of choices that are available and be able to convey this to the person concerned

- plan activities *with* people so that opportunities for choice are available

- listen to and respect people's choices, whether these are negative or positive, and enable them to reconsider if the choice puts them or others at risk of harm

- help people understand the possible outcomes of their choices, deal with any adverse effects and learn from the experience

- support people in taking risks

- balance risk-taking and duty of care

Different kinds of situations demand different kinds of choices, which are influenced by both personal and situational factors. For example:

> Jason has some difficulty with personal hygiene, especially if he hasn't managed to get to the toilet in time, or if he's had difficulty cleaning himself after using the toilet. He needs to be reminded to wash his clothes more often than he would otherwise. However, he has the right to choose whether or not he washes his clothes or continues to wear them as they are.

The challenges facing staff who support Jason could be identified as:

- balancing Jason's personal rights against their duty of care, eg his health and well-being

- trying to understand his level of awareness in relation to the problem

- considering the effects of poor hygiene on Jason's social relationships

- finding creative ways of helping Jason to consider his options and make the decision that is best for him

Effective support for individuals in areas as intimate as continence demands tact, sensitivity, good communication and an awareness of individual rights. Workers need clear guidance and good support from managers. This can be particularly important in situations where they encounter challenging behaviour. McCarthy (1998) tells of a woman whose refusal to wash or change her clothes, despite personal hygiene problems, was her way of exercising choice to gain some control over her life. It's common for us to think of choice as the selection of one from a number of positive options, but opportunities for refusal are equally important and should be respected, as long as they are not placing anyone in danger. McCarthy found that several of the women she interviewed had little choice in managing their own personal hygiene, and were usually told when to have a bath, for example, something they strongly resented.

Encouraging and supporting choice can be particularly challenging when it comes to people with profound and multiple learning disabilities. For instance:

Raymond has profound learning disabilities and cerebral palsy. He uses a wheelchair to get around, pushed by a helper. He can move his arms a bit, and his head, but has very limited movement in his legs. He is doubly incontinent. He doesn't speak but can respond with vocalisation. Raymond has a fairly structured toilet routine as this suits him best. Before Mick, his key worker, takes Raymond to the toilet he asks Raymond if he needs to use the toilet. Raymond is learning to respond with a vocalisation – sometimes it works, sometimes it doesn't. He then tells him where he is taking him, shows him a toilet roll and keeps talking to him to help him relax. When he is on the toilet (where he has support equipment) and while he is being changed, Mick continues to talk soothingly to him to stop him becoming too tense. Mick tries to gauge his mood and match his own response to it. So he jokes with Raymond on some occasions, keeps quiet on others and sometimes plays soft music, depending on how he thinks Raymond is feeling and how tense he is.

What kind of choice is possible for Raymond? Routine is an important part of life and helps us manage and make sense of the world. It can also make a difference between continence and incontinence. Most of us have routine times at which we go to the toilet – an important part of our own health and well-being. However, it's important to ensure that the routine is the *person's* routine and not one imposed by others to ensure the smooth running of the service. You may, like me, have encountered situations where people spend hours sitting on the toilet, with no choice, put there in the hope that they will 'perform'. So is Raymond's routine the best one for him and how can we be sure? Or is it rather that this is the way it's always been done – maybe or maybe not for the best of motives. Have people just made assumptions about him and have these been passed on from worker to worker? Being aware of these possibilities opens up new opportunities for Raymond to make choices. This could mean:

- taking Raymond to the toilet at different times and watching his reaction

- recognising his signs of contentment, preference, approval and discontent and helping him use his own signals for indicating that he wants to go to the toilet

- helping him to develop an awareness of the sensation of being wet or soiled, by drawing his attention to it and enabling him to make an association between this and going to the toilet; by being alert to his signals, they might be able to take him there before he urinates or defecates

- enabling Raymond to choose the music used when he is in the toilet, by watching his reaction to different CDs

Of course, it could be that Raymond's toileting routine *is* one based on his preferences and careful observation of his toilet habits. Even if it is, have all possible opportunities for choice been explored, eg which staff member he prefers to support him, choice of clothes when being changed, choice of pads if he uses them and so on? Staff who are encouraged to adopt an enquiring approach to their own practice in intimate care as well as other areas of work are more likely to become skilled at seeing new possibilities and developing creative responses rather than getting into routines which are more for the benefit of the service than the people who use it.

In order to encourage and support choice effectively, support staff need to be:

- particularly competent in interacting with people who use services

- well informed about continence

- fully informed about individual rights

- aware of their own influence and the influence of the environment

- aware of risk assessment measures

- conversant with the organisation's policies on health and safety, adult protection and care management

Reflection

You might like to think about...

...members of your staff who are particularly skilled in encouraging and supporting staff. What, in particular, makes them so good at doing this? Could this be used to better advantage with other staff?

The importance of good communication in choice-making

Choice and active involvement in continence management hinge upon good communication. In their training pack, *Making it Personal: Providing Intimate and Personal Care for People with Learning Disabilities*, Cambridge and Carnaby (op cit) provide a series of line drawings which can be used both for staff-to-staff discussion and for staff–service user communication and which deal with the range of issues that arise from providing and receiving intimate care, including choice and participation.

Often there is a tendency to get continence support over with as quickly as possible with minimal interaction, which limits opportunities for choice and control for the service user. It is important for staff to take enough time and make full use of the opportunities available to facilitate interaction and encourage choice. This also conveys the message that continence management is a natural part of life and nothing to be ashamed of, and that the person concerned can influence what happens.

The diversity and range of needs mean that communication will vary considerably from one situation to the next. Consider, for example:

> Andy, who is 72, has moderate learning disabilities and has recently had a stroke that has affected his mobility and speech. Previously able to manage his own continence, he now needs assistance with getting to the toilet, using it, managing his clothes and managing personal hygiene.

> Reena, who has severe learning disabilities, has never achieved continence. She needs to be reminded to go to the toilet. She wears continence pads. She communicates using Makaton and some single words that are quite difficult to understand. She lives with her family who work closely with day centre staff.

> Liam, who has profound and multiple learning disabilities, uses a wheelchair and is doubly incontinent. Like Reena, he lives at home, with his mother and older sister.

> Karina, who has stress and urge incontinence following an operation, is currently undergoing continence assessment. She has severe learning disabilities and communicates verbally.

Effective communication with Andy, Liam, Reena and Karina will vary according to their different needs and abilities, although there are some common threads, eg we all communicate with our bodies as well as our voices. It can be helpful to consider separately communication with people who speak and with those who communicate mainly in other ways, as the support needs of each group have particular implications for providing opportunities for choice.

Communicating and encouraging choice with people who communicate verbally

Choice can be encouraged and supported by:

- using symbols, books, photographs and pictures to explain about self-management and encourage choice (the resources section of this book provides examples of easy-read books and leaflets produced for this purpose and also additional sources of information)

- adapting leaflets produced by continence organisations

- planning management strategies with the person concerned, using person-centred approaches, eg concerns, preferred ways of doing things, 'good day–bad day' discussions, graphics

- visiting continence specialists together with the person and helping to mediate the conversation where necessary

- obtaining and explaining information about the various continence aids available and, where possible, the aids themselves; supporting people in trying them out

- encouraging choice in clothing, especially where more suitable, or more fashionable clothes will improve confidence, self-esteem and control

One mother said:

> 'I know that I think sometimes, "My goodness, my daughter doesn't know what it feels like to just wear a pair of pants." Something that I take for granted every day. She's always got this nappy on. And also the practical implications of that as well, like clothing. Often in people with learning

disabilities the incontinence pad is so obvious. You think
there must be something the parent or the carer can do to
minimise this, to get away from this attitude that they are
not that aware of it, so it doesn't matter. Like, for example,
I've spoken to you about this before, that all the trousers
they are making now are these low hipsters, and you don't
want your 21-year-old daughter to have a yard of nappy
showing above it, but at the same time you don't want
them to be dressed in brown crimplene ones out of M&S
that someone in their 50s or 60s would be wearing. I think
clothing is quite a big issue too. You must be guided by
yourself – I wouldn't, for example, want to wear a pair of
close-fitting jeans with a huge sanitary towel. So if you
have the choice to go and get something more discreet,
for someone with a learning disability, that choice is denied
them quite often. Be aware of practical things, but how can
you minimise this person looking different – it's an issue
that's been neglected.'

Communicating and encouraging choice with people who communicate in ways other than through speech

There is a considerable amount of information available about communicating
and building relationships with people who have profound and multiple
disabilities and who don't communicate in words. (Some resources are
listed towards the end of this book.) Effective communication with people
with profound and multiple disabilities requires good observation, the
ability to recognise the individuality of the ways in which different people
communicate and to take the lead from the person. It is important to gather
information about existing patterns of interaction and use these as starting
points for building more advanced communication. The sensitivity of the
communicating partner is highly significant, more so than the abilities of the
person with the learning disability. By building up a comprehensive picture
of a service user's preferred ways of communicating, preferences and dislikes,
and taking into account the situational context and its effect, eg the place,
others present and the person's state of health and well-being, the support
worker is in a much better position to know how to provide opportunities for
choice, to respond and to support decisions. Family carers are particularly
adept in helping support workers build a fuller picture of a service user's
communication, but their expertise is not always capitalised upon. (Bradley
and Ouvry, 1998; Grove et al, 2000; Nind and Hewett, 2001; Wilder et al, 2003)

Techniques which prove useful in encouraging and supporting choice for people with profound and multiple learning disabilities include:

- the use of verbal and physical prompts, eg Makaton, gestures accompanied by simple language to show what you are doing and offer choices

- teaching people specific signs, symbols, pictures or objects related to continence, using them consistently and often and helping people learn how to use them

- the use of referential communication, which works by using an object closely related to a situation to help someone understand better what has happened or is about to happen, eg using a toilet bag as the object of reference for 'bath' or 'shower'; once the person concerned learns to associate the object with the event (which usually takes some time) he or she is then more able to indicate preference as to time, for example, or to express refusal

- using physical contact to develop communication and indicate and support options or choices, eg a light touch on the arm to draw attention, help with reaching out towards something, but only when you're sure that this is the person's intended choice, using touch to help people experience different sensations (cream or talcum powder, for instance) and observing their response

Two publications are particularly useful. *See What I Mean: guidelines to aid understanding of communication by people with severe and profound learning disabilities* (Grove et al, 2000) includes a series of forms for collecting and interpreting information relating to the decision-making process, the communicative abilities of the service user and the process used by the communication partner (staff member or other person). *A Practical Guide to Intensive Interaction* (Nind and Hewett, 2001) gives guidelines on the use of 'intensive interaction', an approach to helping people with severe communication problems learn more about the fundamentals of communication and relationships.

It can often be difficult to be certain that we interpret the communication of people with profound and multiple learning disabilities correctly. There is a need, therefore, to validate a service user's communication by working with family members and other staff to share information and build up a reliable picture of how that person communicates, as well as what helps and hinders communication. The more regular and more prolonged our interaction with the person, the more likely we are to be accurate in our interpretations.

We must also be aware that the responses of people with profound and multiple learning disabilities are idiosyncratic, ie have a meaning that is specific to that person (Porter et al, 2001). Devices such as 'communication passports', 'communication profiles' and 'care books' have proved useful in helping to understand the communication of individuals with profound and multiple learning disabilities and involve them in choice and decision-making. These provide detailed information about the ways in which the person communicates and interacts, and serve as starting points for consultation (Tilstone and Barry, 1998). In most services, more than one person is normally involved in providing support to someone with profound and multiple disabilities, and patterns of work, such as shift systems, can impede communication between different workers and between workers and family carers. Approaches such as these can facilitate the sharing of information between the professionals and family carers who are working together to support the person concerned.

Communication is essential for supporting choice-making but there are other competences staff need to develop. These include:

- becoming a skilled observer

- learning about an individual's patterns of urination and evacuation and planning around this, but doing this sensitively and in discussion with the person concerned or the primary carer

- helping people find out about and consider the relevance of different continence aids

- planning continence management with and not for the person concerned

- ascertaining the person's individual preferences in relation to timing, continence aids and ways of doing things

- following people's individual lead in managing continence – everyone knows their own body best

- understanding that encouraging choice means accepting what the person chooses, with due regard for possible adverse consequences and how to prevent them

- helping the individual, or a carer, access advice from continence specialists, eg continence advisers

- being aware of the different communication roles they play when they are encouraging and supporting choice, eg a listening role is different from an informing role, which in turn differs from the role of helping someone weigh up likely outcomes

It's important also for staff to understand the pressures family carers experience. One mother told me of the difficulties both she and her teenage son are experiencing:

> 'Well, he's got, as I said, no speech at all and it's mostly now that his frustration is getting harder the older he's getting. I don't know if his body is changing, you just don't know. He's not well just now. I don't know what's wrong with him, and he can't tell you – you don't know, it's difficult. He can be quite rough in different things – I think that's all down to frustration, because he's getting big and heavy now – and once I could just lift him to do things with him, but not now. He's too heavy now. I can feel him getting annoyed and it can take like maybe an hour every night with him in a temper, and you don't know what's wrong. We thought of getting the video camera back up ourselves, to get a bit of footage for the doctors – the doctors don't see this problem, they think he's just a perfect child who can't speak, but that's not true. It's getting harder for us, but more for him – the frustration is worse.'

The manager's role in helping staff encourage and support choice

The final section in this chapter explores the implications of previous discussions for you, the manager. It focuses particularly on practices which value and support the work of front-line staff while at the same time encouraging choice and the self-management of continence for people who use services. Most of this will also be relevant to family members, especially where people live at home with their parents or have profound and multiple learning disabilities.

The first point to reflect upon is that choice can only take place in an environment that is supportive for staff, individuals who use services and their families. This is clearly a management responsibility. Cambridge and Carnaby (op cit) remind us that staff are more likely to work effectively if decisions about intimate care are taken jointly. They suggest the establishment of 'working groups' for the exchange of ideas and experiences and to help staff find new and better ways of doing things.

Continence management is not a separate part of life but is affected by, and has an effect on, what is happening in other areas of life. Experience of choice for other purposes will have a positive effect on the self-management of continence. A service which promotes empowerment as an integral element of all practice is in a much stronger position than one which deals with different aspects of practice in a less co-ordinated way. Similarly, services which are already well into person-centred approaches will have service user choice as one of their basic tenets.

The manager's role in encouraging and supporting choice in continence management involves:

- creating a supportive and responsive environment for choice

- providing day-to-day support for staff

- providing training to help staff encourage and support choice

- ensuring that continence management is given appropriate consideration in care plans

- promoting teamwork between individual staff members and between staff, family carers and other professionals

- facilitating reflective practice

- policy development and implementation

- taking due consideration of legal implications and requirements

Creating a supportive environment for choice

This includes:

- a conducive physical environment, eg layout and the use of space (easy access to toilet, bathing and washing facilities, space for changing benches); aids and adaptations (bars round toilets, rollators, hoists); equipment and resources readily available (continence products, suitable chairs)

- an enabling psychological environment, eg ensuring privacy and avoiding intrusion; the language used by staff and individuals who use services (vocabulary, tone and volume); the attitudes and behaviours of staff (supportive and helpful as opposed to insensitive and condemnatory)

- an empowering social environment, eg good relationships between the service user and the staff member requiring help; joint working between the person, relevant staff members and family members (where appropriate); listening rather than telling, assisting rather than doing

Choice is nurtured most effectively in a climate where there is openness and where people are not afraid to seek advice or make mistakes – staff as well as individuals who use services. A service which promotes and supports reflective practice is more likely to find solutions to its own problems and build up expertise than one where people see uncertainty as failure. Confident staff who feel trusted by their managers and who are valued for their contribution to service and service user development are never afraid to seek guidance.

ACTIVITY 2:   **Supporting and promoting choice**

Think about your own service and answer these questions:

In what ways does the ethos and philosophy of the service promote and support choice?

What training do staff get on encouraging and nurturing choice in intimate care?

What are the supports for choice and the barriers to choice in the physical environment?

What are the supports for choice and the barriers to choice in the social environment?

List three things you as a manager could do to extend the opportunities for choice in continence management.

Describe how you will communicate this information to staff.

Day-to-day support for staff

As you know from your own experience, continence is a difficult area for the majority of staff, so ongoing support is crucial. Cambridge and Carnaby (op cit) impress upon us the importance of staff discussions, especially in relation to the more challenging aspects of continence management, such as challenging behaviours and sexual arousal and behaviour. Within their series of line drawings which were referred to earlier, they depict different challenging events, such as sexual arousal, masturbation and inappropriate touching of staff, among other things. These drawings can act as a vehicle for staff discussion and for staff to discuss with individuals who use services and, where appropriate, family carers.

Staff training and reflective practice

Some of the training that staff need to enable them to encourage and support choice will be covered by general training courses, but there may at times be a need for more specialist training. If workers are going to inform people about their options, for example, they need to be clear themselves about what is available and what is possible. They also need to have a sound idea of what people are entitled to. The publication *Essence of Care: Benchmarks for Continence and Bladder and Bowel Care* (op cit) is particularly useful here. Training can be given in different ways: by bringing continence specialists in; by sending individual staff or parents on courses and cascading this information; and by supporting staff to undertake S/NVQ or LDAF training in continence management.

Supervision, given its confidential nature, is an ideal opportunity for facilitating reflective practice in continence management. This is a time when managers can encourage review and reflection and help workers to become more familiar with the complexities surrounding choice, especially the effects of their own more subtle behaviours, eg suggesting a particular choice by the questions they use, showing disapproval in tone of voice or facial expression and conveying distaste for the task. Supervision also provides an opportunity to point staff in the direction of further information, to encourage them to try out more imaginative ways of working and adopt a problem-solving approach to the provision of choice. There is a tendency in all of us to look for prescriptive ways of doing things rather than finding our own solutions. Supported learning, encouraged during supervision sessions, is more likely to enable staff to develop a range of flexible skills and approaches which will prevent them getting into a rut or always looking to other people for solutions. This will also reinforce the value of individual staff contributions to practice and should help maintain motivation.

Continence support for most people involves at least some degree of touching and possibly lifting and moving. Your organisation will have a policy on moving and handling which will have to be followed. Many local authorities and organisations have a policy which does not allow manual handling. Recently, for example, the national news reported on a situation in which a woman with multiple sclerosis had to sleep in her wheelchair for a number of years because of a ban on manual handling. In situations where a manual lift is required, this has to be done by three people, which is very intrusive for the service user concerned. You will no doubt be familiar with the heated debate that surrounds this issue, with people who use services' needs, rights, health and well-being on one side and workers' health and well-being on the other. The following comments from www.communitycare.co.uk reflect the nature of the debate:

'With proper training, monitoring, and risk assessment, yes care workers should be lifting the people they support, if the person prefers being moved manually. Very often being lifted by hoist or similar is uncomfortable, undignified and at times frightening.'

Sue McLellan

'I do not think it right to lift a disabled person unless they are using the correct aid for lifting. I used to lift my son who is disabled and through the years, due to this, I've had trouble with my back and think if I'd had the proper aid then to lift him with may not have suffered the way I do now.'

Caroline Brooker

'There is a reason for no lifting policies – it is to stop severe injuries. Carers are becoming more and more aware that they have rights and do not have to put themselves at risk... We must continue our search for better and more suitable lifting equipment and adaptations that make disabled people feel safe, secure and respected, this should always be a priority, but there are many new items on the market that just keep getting better and better.'

Anonymous

'As the two articles in your feature demonstrate, it is necessary to lift. Hoists are undignified and impossible to use in certain situations. What is needed is: higher staffing levels, more innovation, more time to assess and devise best practice for each individual case. Councils should not ban lifting. Care workers should be medically assessed before working with immobile clients. They should be given appropriate support – including adequate staffing levels.'

Heather Pomroy

One mother of an adult daughter told me:

'I don't know of many parents who don't have some difficulty with their back. They know, I think, that they've only themselves to blame, because most have now got hoists, which I found not particularly helpful – my daughter sits in a moulded wheelchair, very difficult to get round the plinth (it's not pliable). There's a mesh type one now that's used for bathing, which I don't have – I've never had one. I'll now need to look at that because it's very pliable – difficult to get her in and out of the chair – and because it all takes time to do that I think. What you think is, "I think I'll just lift her, lift her on my own." Lots of other parents refer to the hoist as the clothes horse, good for drying the odd towel on, and not much else. You're your own worst enemy.

But I think again that when occupational therapists come out to the house and start looking at hoists and bath aids and aids to be used in the toilet, you're in a domestic situation, it's very difficult – most people's bathrooms aren't that big – and to try and get you the smaller stuff. I've got the smallest type of hoist – a hoist, that's just for domestic use – yet my daughter still gets bumped off the door, you are trying to be so careful. So you think maybe it's safer for her, so you don't use the hoist and you end up with a long-term back problem. So you get into a situation of thinking, well, I have to use this hoist – so it's getting into good habits as well – and I think a lot of parents don't have particularly good habits. Again, when I go out to family centres, or the centre that my daughter went to, there the hoist is used all the time, because that is what they have to do, by law – and when you see that, it looks so quick and easy using the hoist, but when you're in the home situation by yourself – I think it's probably because you're thinking, oh, I've left the potatoes boiling, or the phone's ringing, or someone's at the door – so you can't really compare it to a residential situation or a nursing situation, because there are always so many other things on your mind at the time. So if you're thinking it's going to take you ten minutes, you could lift her in two minutes – it's definitely the time factor.

I'm quite fortunate that my house is fairly adaptable and I've got quite a bit of space in the house. I've felt that when I've gone to other people's homes, like they live in a small flat, I don't know how they manage.

The other thing, of course, if you can think about tracking on the ceiling or that kind of thing – I've never gone down that route, quite simply because your house starts to resemble a hospital ward and I don't really want that – I don't want my house to be like that. I'd rather people came in and it wasn't glaringly obvious that we have someone with a disability in the house – and I think that's fair on my daughter, how she likes it, trying to keep things not so "in your face".'

ACTIVITY 3:   **Both sides of the argument**

Read this extract from the newsletter of the Disabled Living Centres Council (March 2003):

'*The Disability Rights Commission (DRC) has heralded a landmark High Court ruling that, they hope, will end "restrictive local authority blanket bans which refuse to allow care workers to manually lift any disabled or older person from their bath or bed". They called it a humanitarian victory for common sense.*

The blanket bans stem from the over reliance by local authorities on health and safety guidance by the Royal College of Nursing, which was introduced to protect nurses from injury from lifting heavy patients on hospital wards.

Delivering his judgement at the High Court, the Honourable Justice Munby declared that the RCN guidance "is not necessarily an entirely safe guide" and that guidance by the Health and Safety Executive is the most "relevant" to home care situations and the "appropriate" guide, which takes account of disabled people's human rights to dignity, freedom and independence. The DRC, which intervened in the judicial review to give evidence, is aware of similar types of blanket bans in other local authorities.

...The judgement was prompted by the case of two severely disabled women, named as A and B, which marked the end of a five-year battle against East Sussex County Council after it introduced a blanket ban on care workers not to manually lift any disabled or older person. Other equipment, such as hoists, were used but caused pain and the two women asked to be lifted manually, which was refused as it was deemed too 'hazardous' for the care workers. As a result their care package broke down and the parents of A and B were left to do all the lifting, with disregard to their own physical health.

The Court emphasised the need for a balanced approach to the rights of the disabled person and the rights of workers to be protected by health and safety regulations. But the imposing of a blanket ban on manual lifts represented a "no risk" regime rather than seeking to offer independence and dignity to disabled people and minimising risk to workers.

The Court found that: "There may be situations where some manual handling is an inherent feature in what the employee is employed to do."

The judge went on to say "...in the present case, in my judgement, some manual handling is in any view an inherent – and inescapable – feature of the very task for which those who care for A and B are employed".

...This judgement has provoked a large amount of comment amongst all sections of our industry. Here is a selection of reactions from senior figures:

Bert Massie (Chairman of the DRC): "This is a clear victory for thousands of disabled people who have been denied their most basic human rights. There is an obvious need for care workers not to be put at risk of injury in their jobs but this must be balanced with disabled people's independence and quality of life. Blanket bans on lifting all disabled people in the home have had a huge detrimental impact and we urge all local authorities to stop such practices and use Health and Safety guidance that put disabled people's needs back at the heart of the care system."

Michael Mandelstam (quoted in Therapy Weekly*): "It's all about getting the balance right, and the only way you can do this is with good professional assessments. The courts are beginning to say that Article 8 (of the Human Rights directive) invites questions around disabled people's psychological as well as physical integration, and not only their personal needs in their own home, but also their ability to access the wider community."*

> *Carol Bannister (RCN Occupational Health Adviser): "It is important that disabled people are cared for appropriately and are not in pain or discomfort from being lifted. The RCN guidance does not support 'no lifting' policies. The care that people receive should be negotiated on an individual level, based upon the carer and the disabled person's needs. Health and Safety laws require a risk assessment to be undertaken to ensure that health care workers are not harmed by manual handling of patients. The RCN agrees that there needs to be a balanced approach to the rights of the disabled person and the rights of the health care workers to guarantee both parties are protected by health and safety regulations."'*
>
> Identify the dilemmas this raises for you as a manager and suggest ways in which you might deal with these.

Consent for touching

Consent for touching and a choice of how it should be done and by whom are important features of intimate care, but it isn't always possible to reflect on these issues when the task is being carried out. In supervision sessions, managers can encourage workers to reflect on their own performance, the difficulties they might face and their interpretation of people's responses to, and preferences about, touch.

Managers can promote reflective practice in continence care and choice for people with profound and multiple learning disabilities by encouraging workers to ask themselves questions, such as:

- What does N do to show that she likes something?
- What kinds of choices can I offer her, eg the choice of doing things at a slower pace, of letting her do more for herself, of getting more help with things she finds particularly difficult or of using a different type of towel etc?
- How alert am I to her responses about choice?
- What exactly does she do when she's expressing a preference?
- How can I tell my interpretation of her actions is accurate?

A support worker told me:

> 'You need loads of skills. One skill you need a lot, you need respect, listening, communication, understanding, being able to give the right support at the right time, being able to give intimate care respectfully, being able to know when to back off, if you like, so that you don't take away independence.'

Understanding the responses of someone who communicates non-verbally is not easy. The stronger the relationship, the more adept we are at interpreting non-verbal communication, which is one reason why family carers are so valuable in this respect. Undoubtedly, there are times when it is impossible to tell what someone is communicating to you. Bearing in mind that communication breakdown occurs in ordinary everyday interaction with people who communicate in words, as well as non-verbally, we should not be surprised at the challenges. Nor should we ever give up trying to understand or to communicate. Workers with a commitment to developing the strongest possible relationship with the service user will keep trying – and learning – and will succeed much of the time.

Ensuring that continence management is given appropriate consideration in care plans

Services vary considerably in the detail they include on continence management in people's care plans. Sometimes there is the briefest of information, like 'Take Tom to the toilet at four-hour intervals'. You would suspect that services using this approach and this type of language are highly unlikely to be skilled at promoting choice in continence management. Continence management needs to figure explicitly in care plans if it is an issue for the service user. This doesn't mean that this aspect of the plan needs to be shared with everyone providing support. It can be made available on a need-to-know basis and confined to the small number of people most directly involved. Choice should be written in as part of the strategy and should be based, like all other aspects of the plan, on the person's preferences.

Promoting teamwork between individual staff members and between staff, family carers and other professionals to advance choice

This can be tricky, since continence is such a private matter and we need to maintain confidentiality and preserve dignity. Nevertheless, it is important to ensure a consistent approach to choice in continence management, especially where the person concerned has profound and multiple learning disabilities. Sometimes the team will consist only of the service user and a key worker, or a family carer. Cambridge and Carnaby (op cit) acknowledge the many criticisms of key working, but suggest that it has particular merits for the provision of intimate care as it ensures continuity and upholds dignity and privacy.

Teamwork is sometimes better promoted away from the individual care situation, eg through staff discussion, as outlined above. In fact, collective discussions around ways of encouraging and supporting choice are likely to be more productive, since staff have better opportunities to share ideas and experiences while still protecting confidentiality. This type of group activity can stimulate suggestions on how individuals who do not speak express preferences and dislikes, the kinds of support that work best for different individuals and creative ways of enabling choice, all of which can inform practice within the service. These are also ideal opportunities for bringing outside specialists in to inform staff about entitlements in continence care and the wide range of choices available, eg treatments, management strategies, products and equipment and specialist help available. Staff who are well informed are obviously in a much better position to make opportunities for choice available. Often family carers are in a better position to provide information than other professionals. One mother, who works in a continence service told me:

> 'Well, from my experience, when I started off, before I started in the job, I thought that when I was given a product, that was the only product that they had that was available, that could be used. It was only through speaking to other parents that I discovered that they were getting a better quality product, that they were getting pull-ups, they were getting Pampers, they weren't being given these massive big pads which were basically putting my daughter's shape totally out of alignment when she wore her clothes. And that's important as well for her – it's enough for your child to be different, without making them even more different, for things to be more visible. Certainly, now what I do is, if someone comes to my clinic to pick up for their child, I'll get talking to them – I'll maybe need to tell them that I have a special needs child to start off with, and they get a bit friendlier – and I'll ask them how good the products are. I certainly make a point of telling them what other parents get, what is available. That may not be offered to them

unless they push for it. And unfortunately that's quite often.
I realise that everyone works on budgets and really, where
possible, they are given the cheapest product. And the
cheapest product is certainly not always the best product.
That I would actively encourage the parent to go and not
be palmed off, just to go and ask exactly for what their
child needs.'

Policy development and legal considerations

Choice carries risks, obviously. Balancing duty of care and individual rights
and freedoms is not easy. Chapter 4 deals in some detail with organisational
policy and includes legal requirements. For now, it is enough to emphasise
the fact that choice should figure largely in policy documentation about
continence management and should be translated into clear guidance for staff
practice.

Concluding comment

Empowerment of individuals can only occur if they have choice in their lives.
Promoting choice is not something we are particularly good at, especially
when choices are complex or sensitive, or where people have difficulty
with communication. Creative solutions are required at the individual
level and these can feed back into practice within the service as a whole.
Hence, a collective and integrated approach to choice-making in continence
management is important and the manager has a lead role in encouraging
staff to search for this through reflective practice.

Chapter 4

Organisational aspects of managing continence

Introduction

Because of its intimate nature, the vulnerability of the client group and the potential for abuse, the management of continence has particular significance for service managers. Clear policies and effective reporting and recording are essential to good continence management, not only to prevent abuse but also in order to ensure the health and well-being of individuals who use services, safeguard both staff and individuals and promote good practice.

In this final chapter I explore several organisational aspects of continence management and their implications for you as a manager. These include:

- protection from abuse

- consent

- policy development and implementation

- staff training and professional development

- reporting and recording in continence management

- travel and continence management

- multidisciplinary teamwork

Protection from abuse

Protection from abuse is one of the foremost considerations for managers in the management of continence, not least because most support takes place in private and involves physical contact. People with learning disabilities are known to be particularly vulnerable to abuse. Vulnerability stems from several sources: low self-esteem, powerlessness and communication difficulties. They are also less likely to report abuse, because of being afraid, ashamed, feeling guilty or thinking they will not be believed. Many are inexperienced sexually, so are unable to detect potentially abusive situations. Brown et al, in *Towards Better Safeguards: A Handbook for Inspectors and Registration Officers on the Sexual Abuse of Adults with Learning Disabilities* (1996), say it is difficult to get a clear idea of the numbers of people with learning disabilities who have been abused, especially since researchers' estimates vary, depending on definitions used and the nature of questions asked. Despite this, various studies have made it possible to identify patterns in the sexual abuse of adults with learning disabilities. Sexual abuse is more likely to happen in the person's own home or a service setting and the perpetrator most likely to be someone known to the abused person. Almost all perpetrators identified in studies of sexual abuse have been men, many in positions of trust. Men with learning disabilities were often identified as perpetrators. Sexual abuse is often accompanied by emotional abuse, such as threats and intimidation, which makes it even more difficult for people to report it.

Kirklees Committee for the Protection of Vulnerable Adults (2002–03), surveying services within their area, identified people with learning disabilities as the largest group alleged to have experienced abuse, with the commonest type of abuse being physical and the next most common, sexual.

Cambridge and Carnaby (op cit) identify a number of issues managers need to consider in the practice of adult protection, including decisions on lead responsibility for the planning and organisation of intimate care, safeguards in terms of places where such care is provided, the balance of privacy and protection, visibility in supervision and staff appraisal, risk assessment and back-up support in high-risk situations. Brown et al (op cit) identify four models for the prevention of abuse: setting clear standards and values so that staff know exactly what they must do; using strategies that strengthen and empower people who use services, such as self-advocacy, self-assertion, sex education, men's and women's groups; high-quality recruitment and screening procedures to prevent potential offenders being employed; and ensuring that complaints and allegations are always taken seriously, especially as abuse is rarely something that perpetrators commit only once.

White et al (2003) outline several aspects of environments and cultures that facilitate the abuse of people with learning disabilities. Among them are staff perceptions of people with learning disabilities as of a lower status, high staff turnover, frequent staff absence, poor staff training and competence, imbalances of power (both between staff and individuals who use services and between staff and managers) and a controlling organisational climate. Where support workers do not feel valued and have no say in what happens in the service, they are unlikely to value or respect people who use services. Conversely, good management, supportive staff supervision and an environment that promotes accountability have been identified as factors that protect vulnerable people from abuse (Cullen, 1992; Wardhaugh and

Wilding, 1993; Sobsey, 1994; Cambridge, 1999). Cambridge (1999) identifies the relationship between the manager and support staff and the level of competence of the manager as prime determinants of either abuse or support.

In 1998–99, the Department of Health carried out a study of social and health care services for people with learning disabilities in 24 local authorities across England, one aspect of which was protection from abuse. They found that, although there were signs of progress towards improved interagency policies in the prevention, detection and investigation of abuse, there were considerable shortcomings, eg a fifth of authorities had not agreed policies and only half had provided staff training (DoH, 1999a).

Experience has taught many people with learning disabilities to be passive and compliant. This means that they have had few opportunities to assert or protect themselves. Although the onus for protecting them from abuse is on managers and staff, there is also a need to enable them to safeguard themselves. Harper et al (2002) suggest a method known as 'protective behaviours' as particularly useful for this. It is, they say, 'a simple and effective process which enables people to identify and deal with situations in which they do not feel safe' (p.149). The protective behaviours approach is based on the premise that we all have a right to feel safe all of the time and that nothing is so awful that we can't talk to someone about it. People are taught to recognise what feeling safe feels like and how this contrasts with feeling unsafe. They are encouraged to be persistent in their communication and, if no one listens, to keep on trying until someone does. Each person develops a personal support network of trusted and supportive people they can turn to for help. If need be, separate networks can be identified for different places – home and work, for example. Harper et al have used the strategy with individuals with learning disabilities and with groups of both staff and people who use services. They recognise the limitations of the process, especially for people with profound and multiple learning disabilities and acknowledge that many of the ideas aren't new. Nevertheless, they believe it has much to offer to people with learning disabilities in terms of self-protection.

Adult protection is governed by a number of Acts of Parliament, among them the Adults with Incapacity (Scotland) Act 2000, the Care Standards Act 2000, the Human Rights Act 1998 the Data Protection Act 1998 and the National Health Service and Community Care Act 1990, all of which place responsibilities upon local authorities and services. The publication *No Secrets*, issued by the UK government in March 2000 and reviewed in 2002, provides guidance on the development and implementation of multi-agency policies for the protection of vulnerable adults from abuse and is useful for policy development.

Consent

The concept of consent is an important one in continence management. Central government provides guidance about consent in relation to people with learning disabilities and the Scottish Executive does the same in the Adults with Incapacity (Scotland) Act 2000. In continence care, consent has particular relevance for medical intervention, physical contact and the disclosure of personal information. If the person has a welfare guardian under the Adults with Incapacity Act (in Scotland) the welfare guardian must be consulted and has the powers to take decisions on medical interventions.

People are judged able to give consent to medical treatment if they can:

- understand the information provided for them

- understand why the treatment is being proposed

- understand the benefits of the treatment

- understand the likely consequences of not having the treatment

- make a decision based on the above, freely and without duress

Wong et al (1999) highlight the problem of balancing autonomy and protection from harm in situations where someone is thought not to have the capacity to consent to medical treatment, while a survey undertaken by Turner et al (1999) indicates widespread misunderstanding of the law concerning consent. You will also recall from the previous chapter Harris's criticism of the concept of capacity as defined in legislation with the emphasis on intellectual ability to the exclusion of contextual factors such as social and environmental influences.

Williamson and Johnson (2004) point out that consent is seldom as straightforward as guidance documents suggest. As a result of workshops with professionals in mainstream services, these authors developed a flowchart summarising good practice in obtaining consent from people with learning disabilities, based on Department of Health guidance. They highlight in particular the importance of:

- allowing the person enough time to absorb the information

- using signs, gestures, pictures and objects of reference

- creativity in explaining things, of involving carers and support staff

- constantly checking back to make sure the person has understood

- being sure that the decision is the person's own and made without duress

These authors also provide two very useful lists for assessing and supporting understanding: *Signs to look for that show that a person does not understand* and *Strategies to support understanding* (p.49).

ACTIVITY 4:   **Better communication**

Here are the signs Williamson and Johnson (2004) suggest are helpful for seeing that someone does not understand. The person seems to:

- lose concentration

- lose eye contact

- change the subject

- acquiesce – agree with everything you say

- repeat the last thing you said

- fidget, yawn, bite their lip, play with their hands

- appear to become nervous or anxious

- answer in an inappropriate or inaccurate way

What else would you add to this list?

Suggest three strategies staff could use to help people understand better.

Policy development and implementation in continence management

Continence management is an area of support that is all too often invisible, undervalued and under-researched. It is seen as a necessary and unavoidable aspect of care that you have to get on with but don't talk about too much. The potential for abuse – physical, emotional and sexual – is considerable. Clear policy, explicit practice guidelines and appropriate training are therefore particularly important. For the purposes of this discussion I discuss policy under two headings, *process* and *content*, while acknowledging that the two overlap.

The process of policy development

At present, four main problems appear to beset policy relating to intimate care: that it hardly exists, is handed down from 'on high', is so vague as to be of no use for workers or is developed without any input from people who use services, support workers and family carers. In my own work with social care workers I've found considerable variation across services within the same organisation. Cambridge and Carnaby (op cit) found that policy development is often left to the ingenuity and personal commitment of front-line staff and service managers, with little or no support from elsewhere in an organisation. Policy can only work if it's developed in partnership with individuals who use services, front-line staff and family carers, since they are the people with the relevant experience as comments from parents show.

Involving people who use services in policy development

The most important issue for people with learning disabilities is control over what happens to them. Involvement in policy development and implementation makes this more of a reality. Good communication is the key to the process of real involvement. Some of the people who communicate verbally will be able to participate in discussion of the main issues, such as same sex care, privacy, indicating preferences and so on, although discussion will have to be adapted to take account of ability and understanding. From my own experience and that of colleagues I have found the following points helpful in discussion, especially when the subject matter is sensitive.

It is *always* important to allow enough time for discussion to develop and for people to express what they want to say in their own way. Even experienced communicators and support staff often underestimate the time required. I use a rule of thumb which says: if you think you've waited long enough for a response, wait twice as long; if you think you've allowed enough time to explore an issue, allow twice as much time.

It can be easy to overestimate someone's ability to understand or express opinions, especially when they have an apparently good command of spoken language. Supplementary materials, such as easy-read books, pictures and photographs, are often helpful even when people are verbally fluent. These visual aids serve as a reminder of different aspects of a topic, provide opportunities for people to ask questions and can help in communicating an idea or opinion when the person cannot find the words, eg 'It's like that' (pointing to a picture) or 'I don't like this kind of thing'. It's also very easy to underestimate someone's level of understanding, especially if the person has difficulty with verbal expression, so any assumptions always need to be checked out. Visual aids are useful in helping you revise your own assumptions and build up a picture of someone's comprehension.

Some people have a tendency to want to give the 'right' answers, instead of expressing their own opinions, especially when they have had little previous opportunity to say what they think. This often stems from a lack of confidence and the perceived status of the person asking the questions. I find that people resort to quite skilled methods of deflecting or avoiding questions, eg diverting attention, responding to a question with a question, or responding constantly with 'I don't know', especially where they are afraid of making a mistake.

Many staff, even those with considerable experience, are inclined to ask leading questions, eg 'Do you like...?', 'You get annoyed about..., don't you?', 'And then you talked to..., didn't you? And you found that very useful?' These 'closed' questions invite only yes/no answers, except from very skilled communicators who are able to go on to develop the point. Statements such as 'Tell me about...', 'What really makes you annoyed...', 'What happened next...' and so on, are much more likely to elicit fuller information. Some people will need extra help and prompting, of course – 'Anything else?', 'What about...' – but this should only be done when required. Here, too, visual aids can be an invaluable source of support and stimulation.

Context and social climate have a considerable effect on discussion for all of us. Feelings of anxiety, embarrassment and fear of offending people or saying the wrong thing are common. The introduction of a stranger, eg a continence specialist or an occupational therapist can dramatically but often imperceptibly change the social climate, so account must be taken of the effect on a service user.

It can also be difficult for people with learning disabilities to represent their peers, especially when they have had limited experience of doing this. (This is true of many people without learning disabilities as well.) Distancing yourself from your own perceptions and experiences, finding out about other people's views and representing these fairly and accurately are quite complex skills that must be learned and practised. It is important, therefore, not to assume that consultation with one or two people provides an overview of general perceptions and opinions. People who have had experience of key positions in the self-advocacy movement are more likely to be skilled in representing others. Even they, however, with few exceptions, will find it difficult to represent the views of people with profound and multiple learning disabilities.

Usually the most useful way of consulting people who use services with profound and multiple learning disabilities is to get to know them better and find out what works best in practice. This knowledge, and the collective experiences of staff and family carers, provide a good basis for the development of policy and practice guidelines in continence management. We can get a much clearer understanding by just spending time listening to what family carers say, something we aren't always good at in the pressurised lives we live.

Managers can encourage support workers to gather relevant information by:

- using objects of reference that indicate toilet, bath, shower, dressing or undressing and noting variations in responses

- developing skills in observing and interpreting body movements, facial expressions, eye contact or lack of it, particular sounds as indications of discomfort, pleasure, anxiety and fear; this is challenging, as quite subtle signs can change the meaning of what the person is conveying, and is where input from the family carer is essential

- treating all communication – whether sound or body language – as intentional and responding to this, with the understanding that in time the person will begin to make the association between his or her own action and a response which in turn will lead to more intentional communication

- ensuring that they take enough time for interaction with people with more complex needs and building up a cumulative knowledge of preferences and needs

Involving family carers in policy development

Despite some advances in involving family carers, there is still a considerable amount of evidence that they are frequently ignored and undervalued in decision-making and service development (Brett, 2002). Family carers want not just to be consulted but to have their expertise formally recognised and taken notice of in planning, decision-making and service evaluation and development. Having often been on the receiving end of inadequate services and less than sympathetic health professionals, they have valuable insights into the practice of intimate care.

One mother told me of her own experiences:

'Probably my best help came from other parents, who have gone through the same things. Certainly when my daughter was younger, that was my main source of information, parents who had older children and could say I remember when that happened – those are the people you really tend to listen to, and take seriously.

Sometimes with professionals, who are trying to do their very best, but, for example, I can remember my health visitor coming in to me, "I know nothing about children with disabilities – we did a tiny part on it when I was training, maybe you can help me." That will give you an idea.

That was a few years back; they now have specialist health visitors who specialise in supporting parents who have children with special needs. I think that's quite different now from many years ago, with my own daughter, but certainly in my own experience we relied heavily on a network of other parents for the best kind of advice on where to buy something, or what was a good toy, or how they got their child to sleep all night, what was something that was particularly useful, even down to what kind of incontinence garments were available, or what nappies were the best ones, what ones soaked through, a lot of information from what they were actually living with every day.

That's not to say the professionals didn't have ideas. Certainly people like the health visitor and the occupational therapists, who have a lot of professional knowledge – but, again, you know how you sometimes get bombarded with professional people, very young and just out of college, and you're thinking, "Goodness, they've not got any children, never mind children with special needs", that maybe came out a bit cynical – I would say, yes, heavily reliant on other parents, especially for practical things – for what's the best cot, or how much it cost, for where you can get it cheaper.

Social work – I couldn't say they haven't been helpful, they certainly have, but it's been quite sporadic, because social workers change their jobs so often – my daughter's had five different social workers since she was sixteen – and just when you're building a good relationship with someone,

they disappear off to another job and you have to start the
process all over again. And depending on how experienced
the social worker is – I am certainly assertive enough to say,
look, I don't want someone who isn't experienced, I just
don't want to start training someone up again.'

Family carers surveyed by Shearn and Todd (1996) expressed many negative
views concerning the support services they received. Among their concerns
were lack of control, the inflexibility of services and the fact that the timing of
support was dictated by service providers.

Real partnership with families requires what Hogg (1999) describes as
'a radical reorientation of professional perspectives, but [which] fit well
with growing awareness of what true consultation and partnership entails'.
This requires a significant change in the culture of many services. Family
carers value honesty and respect for their opinions, expertise and experience
(DoH, 2001c). Case (2000) found that 'professionals continue to control the
parent–professional relationship, assuming the role of 'expert', rather than
integrating and consulting parents in a negotiated decision-making process'.
Many family members still perceive the power and status of the professionals
as the main stumbling block to real partnerships and feel themselves to
be passive partners without voices, with their main role as providers of
information (Brett, op cit).

Family involvement is particularly important when the person has profound
and multiple learning disabilities, as several writers attest (Brett, 2002;
Hogg and Lambe, 1998; Lambe, 1998). Brett (op cit) proposes the use of an
'alliance model' of disability which represents disability from the perspective
of the person and the principle caregiver. Within this model, partnership
between the carers and the various professionals involved leads to a better
understanding of disability and tackles the oppression and disempowerment
that family carers feel. The social model of disability, she contends, while it is
useful in helping us understand the disabling effects of society, is inadequate
in relation to people with profound disability since it fails to take account of
those who provide support in the person's life. Since family carers are integral
to their relative's communication, the social model may miss the unique voice
of the individual. This has much in common with Harris's (op cit) assertions
in the previous chapter and with person-centred planning.

Although staff should be aware of the importance of involving family carers in
all aspects of service development, they should also be sensitive to those who
are unable to be involved, or whose involvement might be minimal. These are

more likely to be older carers, those who have other caring responsibilities, eg for a spouse or parent, who have chronic or life-limiting illness or who have disabilities that prevent their involvement.

The voices of 'hidden' carers, such as people from minority ethnic cultures, is of particular concern, since many services find it difficult to interact meaningfully with them. Cultural requirements are often misunderstood, stereotypical views prevail and there are often suspicions on both sides. Shah (1998) points out that many families, regardless of their ethnicity, experience feelings of guilt, confusion and disbelief when they have a son or daughter with a learning disability, feelings which are expressed in different ways. Commenting on the conflicting messages on cultural stereotyping, she says, 'perhaps the only firm conclusion that can be drawn from the literature is that extreme caution needs to be exercised when trying to interpret the evidence' (p.198). Many of the services currently available, she contends, are inappropriate or insensitive to the needs of black people and are rejected by families because they are not flexible enough.

There is often a tendency for services to categorise carers and individuals who use services from minority ethnic groups and not make important distinctions, eg Asian carers. Maudslay et al (2003), in a project involving young people with learning disabilities from a south Asian background, found that participants stressed the importance of their religion and culture and that they were fully aware of the differences between their own ethnic group and others from south Asia, eg Pakistani and Bangladeshi. This reminds me of my own experience of working with African Caribbean children in London in the 1970s when one mother complained, saying, 'You people think we're all alike because we come from the Caribbean, but we're not. We're Jamaican, or Trinidadian, just like you are Scottish or English or French.'

Cambridge and Carnaby (2000), point out that confusion about culture can have either positive or negative effects, saying, 'the constructions we have about ethnic differences could result in open communication about how best to provide intimate and personal care for people from different cultures or lead to difficulties associated with personal care being attributed to people's ethnicity or religion' (p.8). We can overcome some of the barriers by providing information that is jargon free and available in relevant languages, using interpreters and advocates where appropriate, implementing training in which staff meet local community groups and learn more about other religions, cultures and lifestyles and ensuring greater flexibility and creativity in services.

The principles on which a support service are based may not be those which are shared by people from other ethnic groups, eg the concepts of empowerment, advocacy and independent living may be incompatible with the values of collectivism and family relationships in some communities. The employment of minority ethnic staff is crucial in services which provide for people from ethnic groups other than white British, although, as Mir et al (2001) point out, we must guard against people being seen both as experts, consulted on all issues about minority ethnic people who use services, and as troublemakers, when they act as advocates. This can bring them into conflict both with other colleagues and with managers.

Reflection

You might like to think about...

...how well the perceptions and views of people who use services and family carers are reflected in your service policies.

...how people who use services and family carers were involved in the development of policies relating to intimate care.

...how people who use services and family carers from minority ethnic groups were involved in the development of policy relating to intimate care.

Policy content and continence management

Essence of Care: Benchmarks for Continence and Bladder and Bowel Care (2001a) is a particularly useful document in developing policy and explicit guidelines for continence management as it encompasses many of the points discussed above. When developing policy and practice guidelines, you are likely to have to consider:

- guidelines on physical, sexual and psychological abuse and on consent to support or treatment, and cross-references to other relevant policy documents such as adult protection, risk management and health and safety procedures

- the relationship and tensions between care planning and person-centred planning and the implications for continence management

- access to resources and mainstream services, eg health services, aids and equipment

- who has overall responsibility for ensuring the implementation of policy and taking the lead in monitoring practice

- staff responsibilities – who should do what and who shouldn't do certain things, eg new staff who haven't yet received training, younger staff, same sex care

- multidisciplinary partnerships

- ways of managing challenging behaviours such as sexual arousal, masturbation, faeces smearing, retention of faeces, physical attacks on staff, sexual harassment of staff

- the role of staff and managers in relation to mainstream professionals

- chronic, acute or life-threatening illness that is connected with continence

- mechanisms for reviewing and updating policy and procedural guidelines

The link between policy and training in continence management

Even if policy is well developed and clear guidelines exist, they can be practically worthless if not backed up by a corresponding programme of training. Training should be ongoing, phased according to workers' needs and experiences, begin at induction and continue as part of each worker's professional development. It should include in-house training, 'whole service' approaches with contributions from outside professionals, support to individual workers during supervision and opportunities for staff discussion and problem-solving activities. This might seem a tall order given the many pressures on staff time and other training needs, but in services for people with profound and multiple disabilities particularly, it can be undertaken alongside other aspects of intimate care, especially since it is an area that requires a considerable time commitment in practice. In other services, such as day centres, colleges, residential settings and supported living environments, there may only be certain people who require support with continence, so there are likely only to be a limited number of staff who require more in-depth training, although everyone should be familiar with policy on continence care. It sometimes happens that an individual staff member has a particular interest in, and aptitude for, intimate care and is keen to develop this area through additional professional development.

One mother I spoke to highlighted the importance of the link between policy and training:

> 'Basically, there should just be specific training in it – personal care shouldn't be left to chance. There should be clear guidelines laid down, and adhered to quite strictly, because one of the things that can happen and has in fact happened to my own daughter was that someone had got a pad and everything laid out for the change, and my daughter had wet the pad immediately, and one of the people left and my daughter fell off the table because there was only one person there, and she had to be hospitalised. And accidents will happen, but with a little bit of forethought, bring two pads with you, just in case that happens, always have her right on the table, think about your preparation, before you actually start, make sure you've got all you need, make sure there are always two people there. If you've got someone who is particularly vulnerable, who is liable to fall off the trolley, if the trolley is right in the middle of the floor and not against one wall, for example, then you have to think of all these kinds of things. And I think it's up to the manager to go over these procedures with every member of staff, make sure they know at all times this is what has to be adhered to, for health and safety, as well as the more kind of emotional side of it and the dignity and respect and all of that – but health and safety is definitely the first priority.'

The Learning Disability Awards Framework has a unit entitled Helping Service Users Manage Continence, which was referred to earlier in this book. The British Institute of Learning Disabilities (BILD) has produced a workbook to support staff undertaking this unit, which you may have obtained along with this reader. Staff who are interested may want to include continence management as part of their S/NVQ.

Reporting and recording in continence management

Recording and reporting are often required in continence management, most commonly in relation to:

- monitoring particular aspects of health and illness, eg monitoring bodily waste

- providing information for medical purposes, eg to a doctor or continence nurse, monitoring bodily waste

- dealing with incidences of abuse or suspected abuse

- describing the needs, wishes and preferences of the individuals who use services or, where appropriate, a family carer, eg in a support plan or care plan

- providing guidance on how to provide the required support

- dealing with critical incidents or accidents, eg falls, mishaps with continence aids or adaptations to toilets or changing facilities

In addition, staff might also need to record or report:

- practice details for care plans, such as the nature of support required by an individual service user and how this can best be provided, which approaches work best, the effectiveness of continence products, etc

- information that is to be shared with colleagues and/or family carers, eg problems with any aspect of continence

- any instances of discrimination towards a service user, eg within mainstream continence or other health services

- any situation that caused particular distress to a service user, eg having an 'accident' in a public place through lack of an accessible toilet, being unable to get the key for a public toilet, having to change someone on the floor in a disabled or public toilet because of unsuitable facilities

- any situation that caused distress to members of the public or that might result in a complaint, eg a service user urinating in public, or being afraid to go into a public toilet on her own and creating a fuss, concern about a colleague's behaviour or response to a service user in public

Procedural guidelines for recording and reporting should provide staff with explicit information about:

- when it is necessary to report or record information

- who to report to

- how to record information, eg forms and formats

- how to record ways in which they can demonstrate that they have followed the necessary procedures, eg safeguarding themselves, the person concerned and other individuals who use services in hazardous situations; providing reassurance and safeguards in situations involving abuse; responding to the perpetrator of the abuse

- recording or reporting their own support needs in difficult situations, eg abuse or challenging behaviour

Some of these guidelines for reporting and recording will be included in other policy documents, eg risk assessment and adult protection policies, but they should also be made explicit in intimate care policy and procedural guidelines.

Travel and continence management

Policy should extend to all situations in which staff provide support, including travel. Continence difficulties can make travel difficult. Journeys usually involve a considerable amount of forward planning. For example:

- planning routes carefully so that there are frequent stops

- helping the person make sure, or staff making sure themselves if the person can't do so, that they have all necessary aids, equipment and spare clothing

- finding out where the disabled toilets and changing facilities are

- reminding the person to use the toilet, or empty or change appliances or aids before embarking on the journey, or staff doing this if the person isn't able to

- checking out where to get help in case of medical emergencies

- when flying, dealing with the constraints of supporting someone in the confined space of aircraft toilets

Incontinence need not constrain people's outside activities if there is adequate planning and proper attention to detail. Practice guidelines should make clear to staff that no one should have their activities curtailed because of incontinence. In situations where there are particular problems, managers will need to provide individual support to the workers involved. Experienced staff members can be particularly helpful to less experienced ones in planning journeys and family carers can provide useful information.

Multidisciplinary teamwork

By its very nature continence management requires support from different professionals. Central government advocates a holistic approach to health care and an integrated approach to continence care. Continence management cannot be divorced from other areas of a person's life. Medical staff may have specialist knowledge about continence, but depend on the collaboration of people with learning disabilities, family carers, support staff and managers in specialist learning disability services for effective use of this knowledge. As Cambridge and Carnaby (op cit) say, 'there is a collective responsibility for all of us involved in services to co-operate in order to ensure that the necessary arrangements and systems for delivering good quality intimate and personal care are in place and that they are used to best advantage (p.19). Health facilitation and health action plans, described in *Valuing People* (op cit), and hand-held health logs (Curtice and Long, 2002) are useful strategies for enabling people with learning disabilities to access better services, geared to individual needs.

Central government policy highlights the importance of high quality multidisciplinary specialist services, with continuity of provision, partnership between agencies and professions and the use of specialist staff to facilitate the work of professionals in mainstream services. The fact that around 80 per cent of support staff have no recognised qualifications or training (Cambridge and Carnaby, op cit) makes specialist continence staff a valuable resource as trainers, as providers of information and resources and in the development of policy. Joint activity with other professionals, as long as it is in the context of an equal partnership, not only informs staff and individuals who use services, but also empowers them through an increase in knowledge and in confidence.

Styring (2003) points out, that since people with learning disabilities often have a multiplicity of needs, a multidisciplinary approach is essential. Multidisciplinary teamwork spans policy development and implementation, training and professional development and all aspects of practice in continence management. Sometimes, multidisciplinary work will involve only the person with learning disabilities, the support worker and one other person, a continence adviser, for example. At other times, such as planning and policy development, several people will be involved. Multidisciplinary working is the root of person-centred planning, since no one person, no matter how knowledgeable, has all the answers. Creative solutions sometimes come from the most unexpected quarters. Care planning and management, key elements in ensuring that people receive appropriate support with continence management, cannot occur unless there is input from all relevant people. Co-ordination is essential for continuity and consistency of care.

Lacey (1998) identifies several challenges to multidisciplinary teamwork, including misunderstanding about the meanings of the words 'collaboration' and 'teamwork'. She draws attention to some of the other stumbling blocks: the sheer numbers of people who might be involved, differences in the way different disciplines operate and differences in perceived status, among other things.

Support staff will be more able to work with people from other disciplines if they:

- are clear about their own roles, eg providing information for particular purposes, advocating, helping the service user to communicate, obtaining information, sharing their own knowledge

- understand the purpose of the collaboration

- are involved from the start

- understand the importance of multidisciplinary teamwork

- are providers of information and have something to contribute, rather than passive recipients of information

- are engaged on joint activity, eg planning, supporting the service user

- can see that the other professionals share their values and philosophies and those promoted by the service

- understand that they can influence and educate the other professionals in the team rather than just learning from them

As a manager, you have a lead role in promoting and effecting multidisciplinary teamwork. This will include:

- identifying the most appropriate people for the team, which means being aware of the people who have expertise in continence care and/or associated areas, eg continence nurse, OT, physiotherapist, community nurse, practice nurse, GP, pharmacist

- being aware of what services are available in your local area for continence care

- being a skilled communicator; above all, this will be about communicating service ethos and values and ensuring that these are upheld but will also involve facilitating communication between members of the team and supporting your own staff in doing this

- becoming informed about people's rights in relation to continence

- ensuring that individuals who use services and family carers are fully involved

- facilitating the involvement of individuals who use services and family carers from minority ethnic groups, with help from supporters from the relevant cultural groups

- knowing where to access relevant information

- facilitating planning and review meetings

- managing the involvement of any critical incidents relating to continence care, such as abuse or serious accident

This doesn't mean, of course, that you need to be an expert in continence care, as well as every other aspect of support. Rather, it's about being clear about your role, knowing where to access the necessary information and when you should delegate some of the tasks to senior members of staff.

Concluding comment

Continence, like other aspects of intimate care, is a neglected area in the lives of people with learning disabilities. Recent initiatives, as described in *The same as you?* and *Valuing People*, point the way to better health care for people with learning disabilities. In addition, there is increasing interest in the continence needs of people with learning disabilities from specialist continence organisations. Taken together, these developments should have a positive effect on the quality of continence care available to people with learning disabilities and enable them to have greater control over this very important area of their own lives. Specialist services for people with learning disabilities have a prime opportunity to make a significant contribution and stimulate ongoing change.

References

Bradley, A. (2002) *Positive Approaches to Communication* Kidderminster: BILD

Bradley, A. and Ouvry, C. (1998) *Better Choices – Fuller Lives* Kidderminster: BILD

Brett, R. (2002) The Experience of Disability from the Perspective of Parents of Children with Profound Impairment: is it time for an alternative model of disability? *Disability & Society* 17, 7, 825–843

Brown, H. et al (1996) *Towards Better Safeguards: A Handbook for Inspectors and Registration Officers on the Sexual Abuse of Adults with Learning Disabilities* Brighton: Pavilion

Cambridge, P. (1999) The first hit: a case study of the physical abuse of people with intellectual disabilities and challenging behaviours in a residential service *Disability and Society* 14, 285–308

Cambridge, P. and Carnaby, S. (2000) *Making It Personal: Providing Intimate and Personal Care for People with Learning Disabilities* Brighton: Pavilion

Carnaby, S. and Cambridge, P. (2002) Getting personal: an exploratory study of intimate and personal care provision for people with profound and multiple intellectual disabilities *Journal of Intellectual Disability Research* 46, 2, 120–132

Case, S. (2000) Refocusing on the parent: what are the social issues for parents of disabled children? *Disability & Society* 15, 271–292

Corbett, J. et al (2003) Health facilitation for people with learning disabilities *British Journal of Community Nursing* 8, 9, 404–410

Cullen, C. (1992) The sexual abuse of people with learning disabilities. Proceedings of the Excellence in Training Conference, University of Dundee, 26 July 1992

Curtice, L. and Long, L. (2002) The health log: developing a health monitoring tool for people with learning disabilities within a community support agency *British Journal of Learning Disabilities* 30, 2, 68–72

Department of Health (1995) *Health of the Nation* London: Department of Health

Department of Health (1998) *Signposts for Success in Commissioning and Providing Health Services for People with Learning Disabilities* London: Department of Health

Department of Health (1999a) *Facing the Facts, Services for People with Learning Disabilities: A Policy Impact Study of Social Care and Health Services* London: Department of Health

Department of Health (1999b) *Once a Day* London: Department of Health

Department of Health (2000a) *Good Practice in Continence Services* London: Department of Health

Department of Health (2000b) *No Secrets* London: Department of Health

Department of Health (2001a) *Essence of Care: Benchmarks for Continence and Bladder and Bowel Care* London: Department of Health

Department of Health (2001b) *Valuing People* London: Department of Health

Department of Health (2001c) *Family Matters: Counting Families In* London: Department of Health

Earnshaw, K. and Betts, A. (2001) Continence and people with learning disabilities *Learning Disability Practice* 4, 2, 33–38

Ghazala, M. et al (2001) *Learning Difficulties and Ethnicity* London: Department of Health

Grove, N. et al (2000) *See What I Mean: Guidelines to Aid Understanding of Communication by People with Severe and Profound Learning Disabilities* Kidderminster: BILD

Harper, G. et al (2002) Protective Behaviours: a useful approach in working with people with learning disabilities *British Journal of Learning Disabilities* 30, 4, 149–152

Harris, J. (2003) Time to make up your mind: why choosing is difficult *British Journal of Learning Disabilities* 31, 3–8

Hogg, J. (1999) People with profound intellectual and multiple disabilities: understanding and realising their needs and those of their carers. Paper prepared for the Scottish Executive Review of Services for People with Learning Disabilities

Hogg, J. and Lambe, L. (1998) *Older People with Learning Disabilities: A review of the literature on residential services and family caregiving* London: The Foundation for People with Learning Disabilities

Huntley, E. and Smith, L. (1999) Long-term follow-up of behavioural treatment for primary encopresis in people with intellectual disability in the community *Journal of Intellectual Disability Research* 43, 484–488

Hutchinson, C. (1998) 'Positive Health: A Collective Responsibility' in Lacey, P. and Ouvry, C. (eds) *People with Profound and Multiple Learning Disabilities: A Collaborative Approach to Meeting Complex Needs* London: David Fulton

Hyams, G. et al (1992) Behavioural continence training in mental handicap: a ten-year follow-up study *Journal of Intellectual Disability Research* 36, 551–558

Kirklees Committee for the Protection of Vulnerable Adults (2002–2003) Annual Report

Lacey, P. (1998) 'Meeting Complex Needs Through Multidisciplinary Teamwork' in Lacey, P. and Ouvry, C. (eds) *People with Profound and Multiple Learning Disabilities: A Collaborative Approach to Meeting Complex Needs* London: David Fulton

Lambe, L. (1998) 'Supporting Families' in Lacey, P. and Ouvry, C. (eds) *People with Profound and Multiple Learning Disabilities: A Collaborative Approach to Meeting Complex Needs* London: David Fulton

Lancioni, G. et al (2001) Treating Encopresis in People with Intellectual Disabilities: A Literature Review *Journal of Applied Research in Intellectual Disabilities* 144, 47–63

Mansell, J. et al (2002) Residential care in the community for adults with intellectual disability: needs, characteristics and services *Journal of Intellectual Disability Research*, 46, 8, 625–633

Marquis, R. and Jackson, R. (2000) Quality of Life and Quality of Service Relationships: experiences of people with disabilities *Disability and Society* 15, 3, 411–425

Maudslay, L. et al (2003) *Aasha: working with young people with a learning difficulty from a south Asian background* London: Skill

McCarthy, M. (1998) Whose Body is it Anyway? Pressures and Control for Women with Learning Disabilities *Disability and Society* 13, 4, 557–574

McNeal, D. M. et al (1983) Symptomatic neurogenic bladder in a cerebral palsied population *Developmental Medicine & Child Neurology* 25, 612–616

Mir, G. et al (2001) *Learning Difficulties and Ethnicity* London: Department of Health

Mobbs, C. et al (2002) An exploration of the community nurse, learning disability, in England *British Journal of Learning Disabilities* 30, 13–18

NHS Scotland (2002)
Promoting Health, Supporting Inclusion
Edinburgh: NHS Scotland

NHS Scotland (2004) *Health Needs Assessment Report: People with Learning Disabilities in Scotland* Edinburgh: NHS Scotland

NHS Scotland (2004) *Quality Indicators – Learning Disabilities* Edinburgh: NHS Scotland

Nind, M. and Hewett, D. (2001) *A Practical Guide to Intensive Interaction* Kidderminster: BILD

O'Brien, J. (1987) 'A guide to lifestyle planning: Using the Activities Catalog to integrate services and natural support systems' in Wilcox, B. and Bellamy, G.T. (eds) *A Comprehensive Guide to the Activities Catalog: An Alternative Curriculum for Youth and Adults with Severe Disabilities* Baltimore: Brookes

Porter, J. et al (2001) Interpreting the communication of people with profound and multiple learning difficulties *British Journal of Learning Disabilities* 29, 12–16

Rigby, D. (2001) Integrated Continence Services *Nursing Standard* 16, 8, 46–52

Roijen, L. E. G. et al (2001) Development of bladder control in children and adolescents with cerebral palsy *Developmental Medicine and Child Neurology* 43, 103–107

Rogers, J. (2001) Fast-track toilet training *Nursing Times Plus* 97, 40, 53–54

Rogers, J. (2002) Solving the enigma: toilet training children with learning disabilities *British Journal of Nursing* 11, 14, 958–965

Scottish Executive (2000) Adults with Incapacity Act (Scotland) 2000 Edinburgh: Scottish Executive

Scottish Executive (2000) *The Same as You?* Edinburgh: Scottish Executive

Shah, R. (1998) 'Addressing Equality in the Provision of Services to Black People with PMLD' in Lacey, P. and Ouvry, C. (eds) *People with Profound and Multiple Learning Disabilities: A Collaborative Approach to Meeting Complex Needs* London: David Fulton

Shearn, J. and Todd, S. (1996) Parents' Perspectives on Support Services *Highlight 7*, Welsh Centre for Learning Disabilities

Smith, L. and Smith, P. (1998) Promoting continence training with people with learning disabilities *Journal Community Nursing* 12 (6)

Sobsey, D. (1994) Sexual abuse in the lives of people with learning disabilities Summary of presentation to NAPSAC AGM, June 1994, *NAPSAC Bulletin* 10, 6–10

Stanley, R. (1997) Treatment of continence in people with learning disabilities *British Journal of Nursing* Jan 9–22, 6 (1) 12–14

Styring, L. (2003) 'Community care: opportunities, challenges and dilemmas' in Markwick, A. and Parrish, A. (eds) *Learning Disabilities, Themes and Perspectives* London: Butterworth Heinemann

Thomas, S. (2000) Good practice in continence services *Nursing Standard* 14, 47, 43–45

Tilstone, C. and Barry, C. (1998) 'Advocacy and Empowerment: what does it mean for pupils and people with PMLD?' in Lacey, P. and Ouvry, C. (eds) *People with Profound and Multiple Learning Disabilities: A Collaborative Approach to Meeting Complex Needs* London: David Fulton

Turner, N. J. et al (1999) Consent to Treatment and the Mentally Incapacitated Adult *Journal of the Royal Society of Medicine* 92, 6, 290–292

Twigg, J. (1998) 'The Medical/Social Boundary' in Allott, M. and Robb, M. (eds) *Understanding Health and Social Care* London: Sage

Von Wendt, L. et al (1990) Development of bowel and bladder control in the mentally retarded *Developmental Medicine and Child Neurology* 32, 515–518

Wardhaugh, J. and Wilding, P. (1993) Towards an explanation of the corruption of care *Critical Social Policy* 37, 4–31

White, C. et al (2003) The identification of environments and cultures that promote the abuse of people with intellectual disabilities: a review of the literature *Journal of Applied Research in Intellectual Disabilities* 16, 1, 1–9

Wilder, J. et al (2003) Behaviour style and interaction between seven children with multiple disabilities and their caregivers *Child: Care, Health and Development* 29, 6, 559–567

Williamson, A. and Johnson, J. (2004) Improving services for people with learning disabilities *Nursing Standard* 18, 24, 43–51

Wong J. G. et al (1999) Capacity to Make Health Care Decisions: its importance in clinical practice *Psychological Medicine* 29, 2, 437–446

Resources

The following information was correct at time of going to press

Organisations dealing with continence and related issues

British Toilet Association
PO Box 17
Winchester SO23 9WL
Tel: 01962 850277

www.britloos.co.uk

Continence Foundation
307 Hatton Square
16 Baldwins Gardens
London EC1N 7RJ
Tel: 020 7404 6875

www.continence-foundation.org.uk

ERIC (Enuresis Resource and Information Centre)
34 Old School House
Britannia Road
Kingswood
Bristol BS15 8DB
Tel: 0845 370 8008

www.eric.org.uk

***In*contact**
United House
North Road
London N7 9DP
Tel: 0870 770 3246

www.incontact.org

Is There An Accessible Loo? (ITAAL)
www.itaal.org.uk

PromoCon
Redbank House
4 St Chad's Street
Cheetham
Manchester M8 8QA
Tel: 0161 834 2001

www.promocon2001.org.uk

Ricability
30 Angel Gate
City Road
London EC1V 2PT
Tel: 020 7427 2460/9

www.ricability.org.uk

Information and advice on clothing

It can be difficult to know where to obtain advice on clothing, especially since fashions change and manufacturers sometimes go out of business or change their products. The best thing to do is to undertake website searches and make use of specialist organisations. PromoCon, for example, can supply an up-to-date list of clothing manufacturers. Log on to:

www.promocon.co.uk

Organisations with expertise in profound and multiple learning disabilities

Mencap
123 Golden Lane
London EC1Y 0RT
Tel: 020 7454 0454

www.mencap.org.uk

PAMIS
White Top Research Unit
Springfield House
15/16 Springfield
University of Dundee
Dundee DD1 4JE
Tel: 01382 345 154

www.dundee.ac.uk/pamis

Profound and Multiple Learning Disabilities Network

www.pmldnetwork.org

Royal National Institute of the Blind
105 Judd Street
London WC1H 9NE
Tel: 020 7388 1266

www.rnib.org.uk

RNIB Northern Ireland
40 Linenhall Street
Belfast BT2 8BA
Tel: 028 9032 9373

RNIB Scotland
Dunedin House
25 Ravelston Terrace
Edinburgh EH4 3TP
Tel: 0131 311 8500

RNIB Cymru
Trident Court
East Moors Road
Cardiff CF24 5TD
Tel: 029 2045 0440

Sense (Head Office)
11–13 Clifton Terrace
Finsbury Park
London N4 3SR
Tel: 020 7272 7774

www.sense.org.uk

Sense Scotland
43 Middlesex Street
Kinning Park
Glasgow G41 1EE
Tel: 0141 429 0294

www.sensescotland.org.uk

Rights organisations

British Council of Disabled People (BCODP)
Litchurch Plaza
Litchurch Lane
Derby DE24 8AA
Tel: 01332 295551

www.bcodp.org.uk

Disability Rights Commission
DRC Helpline
Freepost Mid02164
Stratford-upon-Avon CV37 9BR
Tel: 08457 622 633

www.drc-gb.org

Disability Rights Commission Scotland
www.drc-gb.org/scotland

Disability Rights Commission Wales
www.drc-gb.org/wales

Advice on toilet and bathing equipment

Disabled Living Foundation
380–384 Harrow Road
London W9 2HU
Tel: 0845 130 9177

www.dlf.org.uk

Factsheets provide information and advice and list useful organisations.

Help the Aged
www.helptheaged.org.uk

Regional offices:

207–221 Pentonville Road
London N1 9UZ
Tel: 020 7278 1114

11 Granton Square
Edinburgh EH5 1HX
Tel: 0131 551 6331

12 Cathedral Road
Cardiff CF11 9LJ
Tel: 02920 346 550

Ascot House
Shaftesbury Square
Belfast BT2 7DB
Tel: 02890 230 666

Equipment suppliers
These are only a few of the many suppliers online, chosen because they either supply a useful product or give good links to others who do so.

N & C Phlexicare
www.phlexicare.com

RSD Hygienics Ltd
6 Canvey Close
Wavertree
Liverpool L15 6XA
Tel: 0151 475 0399
www.rsd-hygienics.co.uk

Total Hygiene Ltd
Bank House
182–186 Washway Road
Sale
Cheshire M33 6RN
Tel: 0800 374 076
www.clos-o-mat.com

Suppliers of the Clos-o-Mat automatic toilet which provides 'flushing, washing with warm water and gentle drying with warm air' (manufacturer's description)

www.benefitsnowshop.co.uk
Online shop selling equipment for disabled people

www.creative-healthcare.co.uk
Manufacturers of shower products for disabled people

www.geberit.co.uk
Suppliers of the Geberit shower-toilet – a combination of toilet and bidet which washes and dries the user and also has an air purifier

Magazines

ERIC says – a quarterly support magazine (available from ERIC at the address on p. 101)

*In*contact magazine, produced quarterly (available from the address on p. 101)

Further reading

Arscott, K. et al (1999) Assessing the ability of people with a learning disability to give informed consent to treatment *Psychological Medicine* 29, 6, 1367–75

Button, D. et al (1998) *Continence: Promotion and Management by the Primary Health Care Team: Consensus Guideline* London: Whurr Publishers

Cambridge, P. (1999) The first hit: a case study of the physical abuse of people with learning disabilities and challenging behaviours in a residential service *Disability and Society* 12, 3, 427–453

Cambridge, P. and Carnaby, S. (2000) A personal touch: managing the risks of abuse during intimate and personal care *The Journal of Adult Protection* 2, 4, 4–15

Colley, W. (undated) Constipation-1 Causes and Assessment *Practical Procedures for Nurses*

Department of Health (2001)
Family Matters: Counting Families In
London: Department of Health

Disability Now (2003) Incontinence: did you
know that... *Disability Now* Nov/Dec 22–23

Disabled Living Foundation (2003)
Clothing for continence and incontinence
DLF Factsheet
(available from DLF Tel: 020 7289 6111)

Enuresis (1999) *Bowel and Bladder
Management in Children with Special
Physical Needs: A Guide for Parents*
Bristol: Enuresis

Enuresis (2002) *Bedwetting:
A Guide for Parents* Bristol: Enuresis

ERIC (undated) Positive Approaches
to Enuresis

Gale, E. and Hegarty, J. R. (2000) The use
of touch in caring for people with learning
disability *British Journal of Developmental
Disabilities* 46, 2, 97–108

Grieve, T. (1998) Continence promotion
among children with severe disabilities
Nursing Times 19, 4, 4–5

ITAAL (2001) *The ITAAL Directory
of Accessible Loos In England*
North Wembley: ITAAL

ITAAL (2001) *The Essential Companion to:
The ITAAL Directory of Accessible Loos In
England* North Wembley: ITAAL

Kilbane, J. (1998) Responding to Allegations
of Abuse: Developing a Framework of Staff
Support *ACT Bulletin* October 1998 6–12

Long, L. (1996) Monitoring Client Health in
Talking Sense 42, 4, Winter 1996

McCarthy, M. and Thompson, D. (1996)
Sexual abuse by design: an examination
of the issues in learning disability services
Disability and Society 11, 2, 205–217

Morgan, R. and Dobson, P. (eds) (1996)
*Guidelines on Minimum Standards of
Practice in the Treatment of Enuresis* ERIC

PAMIS (undated) *Abdominal Massage*

PAMIS *Changing Places: Accessible Loos for
All Campaign Pack*

Parker, C. (undated) *Promoting Continence
and Managing Incontinence with People
with Learning Disabilities* PromoCon

PromoCon (undated) *Choosing Products for
Bowel and Bladder Control*

PromoCon (undated) *Toilet Rules OK?*

Richmond, J. (2003) Prevention of
constipation through risk management
Learning Disability Practice 6, 31–38

Rogers, J. (1998) Promoting continence: the
child with special needs *Nursing Standard*
12, 34, 47–55

Shah, R. (1998) 'Addressing equality in
the provision of services to black people
with PMLD' in Lacey, P. and Ouvry, C. (eds)
*People with Profound and Multiple Learning
Disabilities: A Collaborative Approach
to Meeting Complex Needs*
London: David Fulton

The Nursing and Midwifery Practice
Development Unit (undated)
*Continence: adults with urinary dysfunction:
best practice statement* available from,
Elliot House, 8–10 Hillside Crescent,
Edinburgh EH7 5EA

Ware, J. (1996) *Creating a Responsive
Environment for People with Profound
and Multiple Learning Difficulties*
London: David Fulton

Relevant legislation

National Health Service and Community
Care Act 1990
Data Protection Act 1998
Human Rights Act 1998
Care Standards Act 2000
Adults with Incapacity Act (Scotland) 2000

Most commonly used continence aids

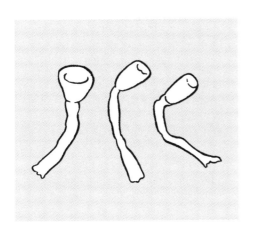

Anal plugs

This is a small foam tampon with a long string attached for easy removal. It is inserted into the back passage to prevent leakage from the bowel and can be left for up to 12 hours. It must be removed to allow bowel movements. It is available on prescription and can be useful for swimming and special occasions. Not everyone finds it comfortable. However, some people have found this aid invaluable when on a long-haul flight – toilets on aeroplanes are not known for being accessible.

Bedding and furniture protection

It is possible to get a range of protective materials for beds, including mattress and pillow covers. Bed pads are used on top of the bottom sheet and placed under the waist and thighs. Some washable pads are designed to hold large amounts of urine and keep the skin dry, thus allowing undisturbed sleep, but the person must sleep naked from the waist down. Urine passes through the top 'feel-dry' surface to the soaker layer and is held there.

Chair pads are also available but are less absorbent than bed pads. They are useful for both ordinary chairs and wheelchairs. These pads might be used in wheelchairs when the person is going on a journey, for example, as a precaution when it might be difficult to find a toilet in time.

Body worn urinals

A body worn urinal might be more suitable if the penis is very small or if the man has a retracted penis. They are normally fitted by a nurse or appliance practitioner who can advise on the most suitable type.

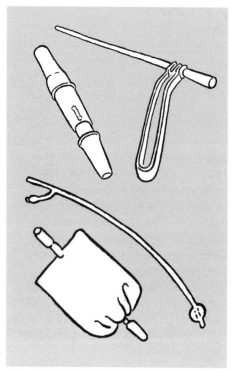

Catheters

A catheter is a fine hollow tube which is inserted into the bladder to drain urine away. Catheters are available only on prescription and must be used on doctor's advice. They can be used either on a temporary basis, eg following surgery, or permanently. There are two types of catheter:

- Intermittent, which the person, or carer, inserts into the bladder and removes several times a day, emptying the contents into a toilet or jug.

- Indwelling, which is usually fitted by a doctor or nurse and is inserted through the urethra or abdomen. This catheter is attached to a drainage bag and emptied through a tap in the bag. The bag can be attached to the leg or worn in a pouch sewn into trousers or skirt. Alternatively, a catheter valve, which is released at regular intervals, may be used instead of a drainage bag.

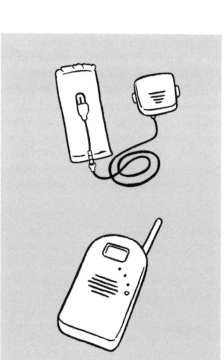

Enuresis alarms

Enuresis alarms can be used to help control accidental urination during sleep. They can be used from the age of five years depending on the level of motivation and the person's ability to manage the alarm independently. There are two kinds of alarm:

- Mini or body-worn alarms have a sensor which can be placed between two pairs of pants or clipped to the outside of the pants and a noise box which is pinned to the pyjama top.

- Bedside or mat alarms have a sensor mat which is placed beneath the lower bedsheet and a noise box which is placed beside the bed.

With both types the noise box sounds when urination begins, causing the person to wake up or 'hold on'. Gradually, the person learns to 'hold on' without the alarm.

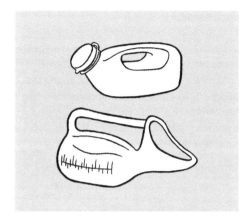

Hand-held urinals

These come in different designs for both men and women, depending on the circumstances in which they are to be used. Most people are familiar with the 'bottle' type urinal used by men after surgery, but there are other kinds.

Also available for both men and women are pocket-size urinals comprising a soft latex bag which folds away into a hard plastic tube. The urinal has a watertight cap and is reusable. It is particularly useful for long journeys or where it is difficult to find a toilet.

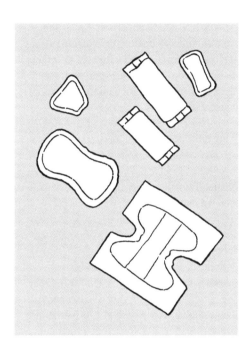

Pads

Pads are the best known and most common continence aids used to protect against leaks. They are worn inside ordinary or adapted pants and are available in different shapes and sizes for children, women and men. Both disposable and washable (reusable) pads are available. Some types of pads are available through local health trusts but others have to be purchased privately. The type of pad which best suits depends on whether the product is for light, moderate or heavy urinary loss or for soiling. The absorbency depends on the type of materials used and not on the size of the pad.

Different pads can be chosen according to different circumstances eg for day or night-time use, short-term use, travelling long or short journeys.

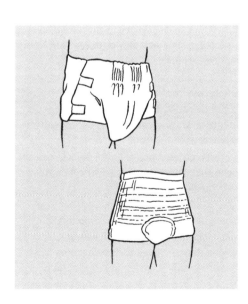

Pants

For men, Y-front pants with a built-in pad or a pouch to hold a pad are suitable for a slight leak or dribble of urine or light staining from the bowel.

For women, there are ordinary looking pants with a built in pad suitable for small amounts of urine or slight staining from the bowel. Pouch pants have a waterproof gusset designed to hold a separate disposable or washable pad. There are also drop-front pants for people who have difficulty with dressing or undressing. Stretch pants in net or cotton fabric are designed to hold disposable or washable pads with waterproof backing.

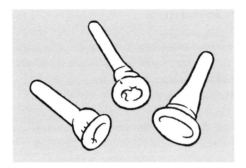

Penile sheaths

This is a soft sleeve which fits over the penis and is attached to a drainage bag. The sheath is normally kept in place with an adhesive strip. Sheaths are available in different sizes and the man must be measured to ensure the correct size – many companies provide measuring kits. Sheaths come in latex and non-latex materials and most can be used only once.

Preventing smells and stains

Used pads and other products should be disposed of immediately, preferably in an outside bin or a disposal unit. Spills and stains should be dealt with immediately and can usually be removed with mild detergent, disinfectant or biological liquid or powder. Most supermarkets stock products that neutralise smells.

(The information above on continence products is adapted from booklets from PromoCon and ERIC. Contact details and further information about these organisations is given above.)

Stoma care

A stoma is an artificial opening from the intestine or in the urinary tract. It is usually the result of bowel surgery (colostomy or ileostomy) or, in the case of a urostomy, a connection between the urinary tract and abdominal wall. Stomas may be temporary or permanent. With colostomy and ileostomy, a special bag is attached to the stoma to collect faeces. Ileostomy bags are drainable and colostomy bags are often closed.

Great care must be taken of a stoma as bowel contents can irritate the skin and result in ulceration and infection. The frequent removal of the bag and seal over the stoma can also cause damage to the skin. It is often necessary to use medicated cream to prevent skin breakdown.

Some people with learning disabilities can, with support and the right sort of information, manage their own stoma bags, but others will need a great deal of help. Those responsible for supporting someone with a stoma require special training which will be provided by the local stoma nurse.

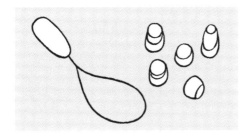

Vaginal cones

These are designed to help with pelvic floor exercises. They come in different weights and are inserted into the vagina for short periods once or twice a day, the lightest weight first, then gradually building up to the heaviest. The muscles tighten to hold in the cones and the exercise helps to strengthen the muscles.

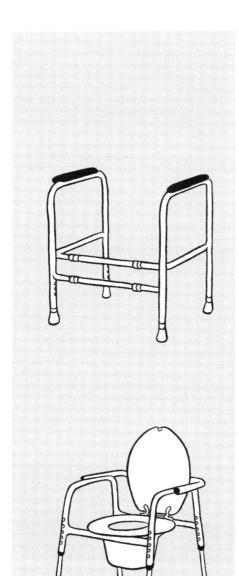

Adaptations for toilets

A good seating position, where the person feels safe, secure and comfortable, is essential for the proper emptying of bowel and bladder. Often, people sit on the edge of the toilet and rush to get off. This can result in poor toilet habits and the inability to empty the bowel and bladder completely, sometimes causing infections.

There are many products available which can help adults feel safe on the toilet and sit properly. These include:

- grab rails which can be attached to the walls to help people get up from the toilet

- rails which are placed around the toilet and give support on three sides, both for sitting down on the toilet and getting up – these rails can be free standing or can be fixed to the floor; fixed rails are not suitable for wheelchair users as they block access; great care must be taken in using free standing rails to avoid falls

- raised seats to increase the height of the toilet

- rails with raised seats

- 'commode seats' which fit over the toilet and support people who have difficulty sitting unaided

Commodes are also useful in situations where people cannot get to the toilet in time, where the toilet is inaccessible or where there are problems finding one, eg when someone is away from home. Portable commodes are useful for travel.

'Shower toilets' flush, then wash and dry the person's genital area, so are extremely useful both in preserving the dignity of the service user and cutting down on tasks for staff.